PRAISE FOR *LIFE AFTER THE DIAGNOSIS*

"While sometimes painful to read, this book is nonetheless a valuable resource guide for patients, their families and their caregivers. Much of this would have been helpful to our family as my husband began his treatment for lymphoma, and then continued it for MDS and, finally, AML. Dr. Pantilat offers refreshing and practical recommendations, wisdom and compassionate support for those facing life after the diagnosis of a serious illness. This book is also a critical endorsement for palliative care at the onset of a life-threatening disease."

—ANN RICHARDSON BERKEY, CEO, The Berkey Group

"This inspirational book is infused with both the science and art of medicine providing a valuable guide for patients and their families to navigate the complex journey of living with a life limiting illness. It is a celebration of both life and death."

—PATRICIA M. DAVIDSON, RN, PhD, FAAN, Dean and Professor, Johns Hopkins University School of Nursing

"While on a journey through serious illness, we would all hope to receive empathy and compassion, knowing that affecting a cure alone is not the only treatment in the art of healing. Dr. Steve Pantilat has compiled a straightforward, sensitive and honest guide, helping to demystify the healthcare system and change the paradigm for patients, their families, and the providers who care for them. As a husband and father, I appreciate insight and guidance on how to navigate the experience from such a compassionate and caring palliative care physician. I wish this book would have been available to my family, as we were guiding my parents through their serious illnesses."

—MARK GANZ, President and CEO,
Cambia Health Solutions

"I am so grateful to Dr. Steve Pantilat for writing this wonderful book. Though he has personally eased the suffering of many thousands of patients (including my own father in his final days), the book allows him to amplify his message for the benefit of the world at large. As a physician, I am terribly grateful to have this resource to offer patients, to help ease their anxiety and prevent needless suffering for themselves and their families. I would recommend that everyone read this book, so we will be ready and prepared for the times we are faced with difficult medical news, either for ourselves or our loved ones. I will be a better doctor, and a better patient and family member, as a result of the advice in this book!"

—TRICIA HELLMAN GIBBS, MD

"My mother was lucky enough to have Dr. Pantilat's palliative medical care in the last six months of her life. In this book, I can hear his humane, pragmatic voice saying, 'Your wishes will be respected and your suffering will be lessened.' I'm glad other families can benefit as we did from his wisdom and deep experience with serious illness."

—JORDAN GOLDSTEIN, CLPF

"As a physician and a former caregiver to my late husband, I adored this wise and comforting book. I will recommend it to patients, friends, anyone facing a life-changing illness. An empowering resource for living better and longer."

—LUCY KALANITHI, MD, FACP, Clinical Assistant Professor of Medicine, Stanford University School of Medicine

"When families are confronted with a difficult disease, it can shake them to the core. Dr. Pantilat's *Life after the Diagnosis* is an essential guide that helps equip patients and caregivers with the tools they need and the words to use to get the kind of compassionate care they want. Weaving together professional advice and personal experience, this book reassuringly answers the call for having a doctor in the house. It's the perfect book to give or get, providing a roadmap for families to navigate the complexities of our health care system while also giving practical tips for identifying the individual's personal priorities so the patient's quality of life remains at the forefront. Dr. Pantilat's shared wisdom feels like having the doctor you want right in your own family, ready to answer your urgent call. This book powerfully recognizes that the art of healing stretches beyond the limits of medical dogma to also embrace care focused on joy, dignity, and relishing the moments."

—REBECCA KIRCH, Executive Vice President for Healthcare Quality and Value National, Patient Advocate Foundation

"During the times of uncertainty and fear that follow a serious diagnosis, this book arrives like a guardian angel. From the importance of finding the right doctor (and how to do that) to taking control back from a sometimes impenetrable health care system, this practical and essential guide is the best of company on the journey. I will recommend it to all my patients, and will keep it close to hand for me and my family too."

—DIANE E. MEIER, MD, Director, Center to Advance Palliative Care

"An invaluable book for those struggling to live well with an incurable disease, written by a doctor's doctor—the sort that fellow physicians seek out for their own care. Short of having him at your side, this is the next best thing."

—ABRAHAM VERGHESE MD, Professor and Vice Chair, Stanford University Department of Medicine

"In addition to being one of the world's most influential and admired palliative care physicians, Steve Pantilat is the doctor we'd all love to have if someone we cared about received an awful diagnosis. In *Life after the Diagnosis*, Pantilat's experience, plain-spokenness, wisdom, and compassion are on fully display, making this the go-to resource for patients and family members grappling with what to do after the doctor says, 'I'm afraid I've got bad news . . .'"

—ROBERT M. WACHTER, MD, Professor and Interim Chairman, Dept. of Medicine Chief, Division of Hospital Medicine Marc and Lynne Benioff Endowed Chair

life
after
the
diagnosis

EXPERT ADVICE
FOR LIVING WELL WITH SERIOUS ILLNESS
FOR PATIENTS AND CAREGIVERS

Steven Z. Pantilat, M.D.

Da Capo
LIFE
LONG

DESIGNED BY LINDA MARK
Set in 11 point Berling LT Std by Perseus Books

Cataloging-in-Publication data for this book is available from the Library of Congress.

First Da Capo Press edition 2017
ISBN: 978-0-7382-1938-7 (paperback)
ISBN: 978-0-7382-1954-7 (e-book)

Published by Da Capo Press, an imprint of Perseus Books, LLC, a subsidiary of Hachette Book Group, Inc.
www.dacapopress.com

Da Capo Press books are available at special discounts for bulk purchases in the U.S. by corporations, institutions, and other organizations. For more information, please contact the Special Markets Department at Perseus Books, 2300 Chestnut Street, Suite 200, Philadelphia, PA, 19103, or call (800) 810-4145, ext. 5000, or e-mail special.markets@perseusbooks.com.

LSC-C
10 9 8 7 6 5 4 3 2

To my parents, Sara and Yoav Pantilat,
who taught me the art of living well, and to
my wife, Cindy, and my boys, Yoav, Ben, and Adam,
who teach me about the beauty of life every day.

CONTENTS

PART III: looking ahead

INTRODUCTION

VIRTUALLY EVERY DAY, I GET CALLS AND EMAILS FROM colleagues, other doctors, friends, and strangers. A loved one has cancer, heart failure, dementia; they're in pain, nauseated, not eating; the doctors want to operate, step up chemo, or insert a pacemaker or a feeding tube, bring in hospice. Their hearts are breaking. They're confused, at a loss. They're concerned about their loved ones, but they don't know what to do. They need help.

I listen, share my experience and expertise, offer advice, and try to help. I wish I could do the same for more people. Since I can't personally talk to everyone, I've written this book— to give others the same information, support, and guidance I give to patients, patients' families, colleagues, students, and others who contact me.

If you or a loved one is suffering from a serious illness, I'm sincerely sorry for the difficult journey that lies ahead. I understand how hard it can be, the heartache, uncertainty, and fear. I'm sorry for the pain, torment, and hopelessness you may feel.

Although it may seem impossible to you now, I want to assure you that your journey can be made easier, less painful, more dignified, and more comfortable. Your pain can ease and you can enjoy better times. That's why I've written this book. I want to help you get through your illness and live life to its fullest.

Before we go any further, let me introduce myself and tell you why I'm qualified to write this book. I'm a physician who is a distinguished professor at the University of California, San Francisco, where I specialize in treating patients with serious medical illnesses. I'm a pioneer and an acknowledged authority in the emerging medical field called "palliative care," which focuses on improving the lives of seriously ill people.

Briefly put, palliative care is dedicated to giving patients relief from their pain, stress, and discomfort in ways that improve the quality of life for both patients and their loved ones. Our main goal is to help patients have the best possible quality of life for as long as possible—to live better and longer. That's also the objective of this book.

Over the past twenty-seven years, I have treated thousands of patients with serious illness and conducted extensive research on treating those patients as well as people approaching the end of life. I've also taught medical students, physicians, nurses, social workers, chaplains, and hospital staff members about palliative care and founded a network that is helping to improve palliative care services nationwide.

Shortly after I began writing this book, my mother was diagnosed with inoperable lung cancer, from which she subsequently died. I've also treated and been at the bedside of other family members, close friends, and colleagues who were seriously ill. As a physician, a son, and a friend, I've gone through the anguish that the loved ones of seriously ill people endure. I've experienced the range and intensity of emotions they feel.

The impact of those experiences is always with me and is reinforced every day.

THE DILEMMA

Serious illness is awful, horrible; there's no way to sugarcoat or minimize it. When I talk about serious illness, I mean cancer, heart failure, chronic lung disease including emphysema, cirrhosis, kidney failure, dementia, stroke, Parkinson's disease, amyotrophic lateral sclerosis (ALS), and others. When such an illness strikes, it hits us hard. The impact is shocking, confusing, and depressing. It can devastate both patients and their loved ones. When an illness is long lasting, it disrupts our lives and drains our emotions, energy, and finances. It makes it hard for us to keep ourselves and our lives together.

Serious illness changes everything. It casts us into new and mysterious territory, somewhere we never wanted to go and know little or nothing about. During serious illness, we see everything differently. Our awareness heightens, and we realize that the risks are greater, the stakes are higher, and the time is shorter. The decisions we must make are harder, more elusive.

When we or our loved ones become seriously ill, many of us don't know where to turn, the questions to ask, or the actions to take. Some of us become paralyzed and fail to act, and others charge ahead and make rash decisions. Many may not be able to completely grasp what's happening, the full meaning of the news they received, and all the medical implications that might be involved.

Simply put, when we are diagnosed with a serious medical condition, we don't have, or can't digest, all the information we need. And we're not at our best. We're upset, scared, and feeling extremely vulnerable. Even though we're reeling, our minds are blurred, and we don't have all the facts, we have to move forward. We have to make decisions—critical decisions—on matters we don't want to face and don't feel equipped to make. We face a steep, daunting learning curve and don't know where to start. *Life after the Diagnosis* tells you where to start and how to proceed.

LIFE AND LIVING

This is a book about life and how to live. Although it's written for people with serious illnesses and those who care about them, it's not a book about dying and death. Instead, it's intended to help clear the fog, provide direction, be a resource, and give seriously ill people, their loved ones, and all caregivers a blueprint to follow during difficult and emotionally wrenching times.

The pages that follow explain that all isn't lost and that you and your loved ones can make the most of your time. They also identify the support you can get and the actions you can take, and they point out that you don't have to stand by helplessly. This book encourages you to be with others and get help, not to withdraw and be alone. During serious illness, you can do a great deal to make your situation better and lead a productive, satisfying, high-quality life.

This book is practical and information intensive. It's a clear, straightforward guide that shows you how to move through your illness in the best possible way: how to live with dignity and be as comfortable and productive as possible for as long as possible—a goal we all share regardless of our present health. It explains the options and what they entail, and states specifically what you can do. In these pages you will find the information you need to make the best, most informed decisions.

CONCLUSION

Helping seriously ill people and their families is my passion; it's my mission, my life's work. Through my career, I've gained invaluable knowledge, unique insights, and special inside information that I want to pass along. Now, I want to share with you, and people everywhere, the same clear, straightforward advice I've given to thousands of patients and to my family, friends, and colleagues—advice that I know will help. My mission is to help you live well after the diagnosis.

The most important lesson I've learned in working with seriously ill people is that our time is limited and precious. Each day, that lesson becomes more powerful and meaningful to me. The message of this book is to make every moment count. Treasure your time and spend as much of it as you can doing what you love with those you love—do it while you can.

Thank you for reading this book. I hope it helps you.

Please feel free to contact me at www.lifeafterthediagnosis .com/comments with your questions, comments, ideas, and personal stories.

Steven Z. Pantilat, MD
San Francisco, CA

AUTHOR'S NOTE

STORIES ARE ESSENTIAL TO MEDICINE. I HAVE LEARNED the practice and art of medicine from the experiences of my patients and their families, and I share their stories to shed light on the challenges to and opportunities for living well with serious illness. The names, ages, medical details, family relationships, and identifying characteristics of all patients have been changed to protect their privacy and confidentiality. Any resemblance to any particular individual is purely coincidence.

PART I

first steps after the diagnosis

chapter one

BAD NEWS, NOW WHAT?

"I'M SORRY TO HAVE TO TELL YOU . . ."

"The biopsy shows cancer."

"It's a stroke."

"You had a major heart attack."

"It's Alzheimer's."

"The cancer is back."

"You have ALS—Lou Gehrig's disease."

Few things are worse than getting bad medical news. It's devastating to learn that you or a loved one has a serious, life-threatening illness or that a condition that was in remission has returned. Bad health news is shocking and can overwhelm you, even when you think you're prepared for it, even when you sense it coming. When you get bad news, you may think that your life has ended, but it hasn't! You will still enjoy many good times and experiences.

When you get bad news, moving forward is never easy, but it's crucial and definitely possible. How you deal with bad medical news may not cure you or make your illness disappear, but it can help you make the most of a rotten situation. Dealing with bad news is the first step forward in reclaiming your life.

> *"Hope is not found in a way out but a way through."*
> —ROBERT FROST

The moment you receive bad news, you see your life differently. You think in terms of before and after your diagnosis. You say, "This is the way I was before—this is how I am now." Bad news gives you a new reality. You know that your life will *never* be the same. The fact is that something massive has moved front and center—it dominates your mind and colors every aspect of your existence. It may compel you to alter your perspective, reexamine your goals, set new priorities, make plans, and change how you act.

Bad news comes in many forms and affects us differently. For each of us, it makes different demands, has different time frames, and moves at different speeds. And although it initially may feel that way, bad news doesn't mean that your life is over or that your world will immediately be turned upside down. Take dementia for example. When people learn that they have dementia, their minds flood with questions and worries about the future, but they usually don't have to make sweeping, life-altering changes overnight. As their dementia progresses, they will have to adapt and adjust, but most of them will still be able to function in many areas for years.

Similarly, with treatment, medications, and lifestyle changes, most people with heart disease can stay active and hardly miss a beat. In contrast, other illnesses, such as cancer, often demand urgent action. With a cancer diagnosis, you may not be able to wait; you may need to quickly make changes that will put your life on hold. Usually, people with cancer can safely wait a few days or even a few weeks to start treatment, but ultimately they may have to drop everything and begin a course of chemotherapy or radiation that can have many draining side effects and profoundly impact their life.

WHAT TO DO

Bad medical news doesn't have to completely shut you down. When you get bad news:

> Take time to deal with your feelings—acknowledge them and let the news sink in. Don't make any major decisions until your head stops spinning and your mind clears.
> Then, look ahead. Think in terms of what you need to do now, today, this week or next. Looking too far ahead can overwhelm and paralyze you. So identify the decisions that you need to make now and those that can wait.
> Learn about your condition, speak to people, get referrals, and find out who provides the most expert medical care.
> Identify the best doctors, hospitals, and clinics, and the medications, procedures, and treatment options.
> Plan. In consultation with your doctors, create a plan of action and a treatment plan. Then identify what you have to do and the steps you need to take. Planning won't change the reality of your diagnosis, but it can change how you, your friends, and your family feel about and deal with your illness. I'll discuss this in greater detail in the following chapters.

> Each time bad news knocks you down—and it will probably knock you down more than once—take a moment, gather yourself, and develop a new plan to overcome the setbacks and move on. A plan can energize you, change your focus, and help you get back up and move forward. You can always do something to try to make things better.

HEARING BAD NEWS

Everyone reacts differently to bad news. Some people are more sensitive and take it hard. They may go to pieces and find they can barely function. Others are stoic, philosophical, and practical. While they put on a brave face, they may ache inside. Reactions can also be mixed, inconsistent, and extreme. No reaction is wrong; all responses are normal. Expect emotional ups and downs, intense and quickly changing feelings. One minute you may find yourself crying, the next you're on the phone with your insurance company to confirm that a certain doctor is part of your network.

When you receive bad news, your brain may freeze and you may not hear or understand anything else that's said. While your doctor continues explaining, your mind may be in such shock that you can't listen or comprehend. You may be so thrown or worried about your fate that you can't concentrate on anything that's said. Your doctor's words don't register; all you hear is "Wah wah wah wah," like when grown-ups speak in the classic Charlie Brown TV specials.

Upon hearing bad news, don't be surprised if you think the worst. Your mind may go directly to death and dying, as it did for my patient Richard.

At eighty-two, Richard was robust and seemed to be in good health. He lived at home with his daughter, still drove, was physically active, and had all his faculties. One morning Richard awoke with excruciating pain in his right hip and couldn't walk. His daughter called an ambulance that took him to the emergency room. When X-rays of his hip proved negative for a fracture, Richard was given a CT scan to see if there was a small hip fracture that the X-ray had missed. The CT scan failed to show a reason for his hip pain, but it revealed two suspicious masses in his liver that were completely unsuspected and not thought to be related to his hip pain. Richard's pain got better and he went home. A biopsy later that week showed that Richard had colon cancer that had spread to his liver.

The next day, Richard and his daughter came to my office for his biopsy results. "I'm sorry to have to tell you this," I said, "but the biopsy shows that you have cancer, colon cancer, that has spread to your liver." I then stopped speaking. For a minute or so, Richard sat expressionless, saying nothing. Then he asked, "So, Doctor Pantilat, tell me, how long do I have? Am I going to die?"

"This is serious," I said, "and it looks like we're not going to be able to make it completely go away. It may well be the illness that ends your life."

"How long do I have?" Richard asked.

We talked about treatment options, the probabilities, and the risks. I told him that I thought he had at least a year and maybe more if chemo worked. As we spoke, I could see that Richard was visibly relieved. "When you told me I had cancer," Richard said, "I assumed that I only had two or three weeks to live."

Although the news was still bad, our conversation enabled Richard to voice his concerns, learn more about his condition, and find out what could be in store. It also gave him better news than he had imagined when he first heard the diagnosis, which lifted his spirits and gave him hope.

WHAT TO DO

Don't leave anything to your imagination. Ask questions; get the complete and accurate picture. Learn as much as you can. Sometimes the truth, as it was for Richard, will not be as bad as you imagine. Don't try to guess what your doctor means, and don't be afraid you will look stupid or take up too much of your doctor's time. Instead of trying to infer what your doctor is actually saying:

› Ask explicit questions to pin your doctor down. If you're confused or don't understand, ask him or her to explain. And be sure you fully understand the answer. If it still isn't clear, ask until you understand. No question is wrong or inappropriate.

› If you can't follow what the doctor says or the news he or she gives you isn't clear, signal the doctor to stop. Hold up your hand, tell the doctor to wait, point out what you don't understand, and ask him or her to explain. If you need time to digest what you were just told, say so. During the pause, think about the questions you want to ask. And if you can't think of any questions or even concentrate, which is often the case, tell the doctor that you're going to have to stop now and come back at a later time when you've had the chance to absorb it all and think.

I find that when I'm a patient, I don't always understand everything my physician says. If I, a medical professional, can be confused, people who don't have medical backgrounds also can be confused. Like me, they have the right to, and should, insist on clear explanations.

> › If you have doubts or questions about your diagnosis that your doctor can't satisfactorily resolve, get another opinion. Get the names of experts and consult them.
> › Ask your doctor if he or she can recommend websites that you can visit or materials that you can read to learn more about your condition and what it may entail.

A word about the Internet, which I'll address in greater depth in the next chapter. Websites that post information from people with your condition can be extremely helpful. They can help you gain insight into your illness and what it's like to go through it. Although many excellent medical websites exist, the Internet also contains lots of very bad health information. Predators also abound online who hope to make a buck by offering miracle cures to seriously ill people. So be careful; verify all information, promises, and claims you find on the Internet.

> › If you have an important doctor's appointment during which you may be given bad news or will be discussing treatment options, bring someone with you. That person may be able to listen and remember the news more clearly and accurately and be able to help and comfort you.
> › Consider writing down what your doctor says. Then read what you've written back to your doctor to verify that you understood it correctly. Say, "Let me make sure I got this right." You can also bring an audio recorder to tape

the meeting so you can listen to it again. Just be sure to get the doctor's permission before you start recording. If you need to, download a smartphone audio-recording app such as iPhone PMC Recorder or Smart Voice Recorder (for Android).

› Don't be hard on yourself because of how you respond.

Some people don't ask questions because they're afraid to hear the answers. They often imagine the worst or try to ignore their problems. Ask questions. The bad news you receive may not be as bad as you fear. And even if it is, that information will enable you to do something about it as opposed to not knowing, which will keep you in the dark. When you act promptly, it can have a positive impact. If you ignore the problem and later decide to act, it may be too late.

If you would rather not ask questions, you have other options. You can simply trust the doctor to do what's best, or have a loved one or friend speak with your doctor on your behalf. Patients frequently ask me to talk with their wives, husbands, sons, daughters, nieces, or friends whom they want to make decisions for them. The best approach is the one that works for you. And if you subsequently decide that you want to get information directly from the doctor, you can always change your mind.

The patient-doctor relationship is a two-way street. Essentially, it's just an interaction between two human beings. Patients tend to defer to doctors. As a result, many don't fully question doctors when they receive horrible news, which is understandable. Although it's essential to ask questions when you get bad news, it's hard. So take enough time to clear your mind and formulate questions so you can get the information you need to make the best decisions on how to proceed. You may have to schedule another visit to ask your questions.

I suggest to patients that they write their questions down when they think of them so they can ask them when we meet. Carry a pad, notebook, or smartphone with you to note whatever comes to mind. I do the same before I visit my doctor and before we see my children's pediatrician. I started this practice after I left a pediatrician's office yet again with many questions unanswered. I figured that I get only one shot a year to ask the pediatrician questions and realized that I needed to be prepared to make the most of that visit. If it makes sense to write a list of the questions you want to ask during a healthy child's annual checkup, it's even more important to make a similar list before your visits regarding serious illness.

SLAYING DRAGONS AND MAKING PLANS

Serious illness usually involves a series of events, and when you're seriously ill, your emotions bounce around. Periods of calm may mix with moments of terror. Once you slay one dragon, another may appear. You may be able to slay some dragons, but some you can't. You may even learn to live with a few. That's why it's so important to have a plan. Often, what the plan is isn't as important as the fact that you have one.

Shortly after I began writing this book, my mother was diagnosed with incurable lung cancer. From the outset, every piece of news we got about her condition was bad. Whenever developments could be either good or bad, they were invariably bad—worse than we hoped. Here are just some of the setbacks we received. We hoped that:

> The rib pain my mother had for six weeks was just a strain—it wasn't.

> The spot on my mother's chest X-ray was nothing—it was.
> She didn't have lung cancer—she did.
> My mother had a treatable form of lung cancer—she didn't.
> She wouldn't have many complications—she did.
> Her complications would be mild—they were draining and debilitating.

One complication was a nasty bladder infection that made my mother very uncomfortable. As part of her treatment, a catheter was inserted. Although the catheter was intended to give her some relief, it added to her pain and discomfort. During one of my visits she told me, "Oh, if I could only get rid of this bladder infection and this catheter, I'd be great."

My first reaction was that her bladder problem was nothing, compared with her cancer. At the time, I was searching for new treatments for her cancer and not worried about a simple bladder infection. In the big picture, it seemed like a tiny bump, a distraction, a trivial issue. But I soon realized that her infection and the catheter were a dragon to her—and one we could slay. Her comfort was paramount. Something I considered a nuisance, especially when compared to her lung cancer, was causing her great pain. Addressing her bladder infection quickly and decisively and having the nurse remove the catheter was a clear, concrete plan that helped my mom feel better.

PUTTING IT IN PERSPECTIVE

Let's face it, bad medical news stinks; it's difficult to handle and can feel extremely unfair. Some people are struck far too early, and many patients and their loved ones have to suffer through long, excruciating sieges.

Although getting bad news is horrible, it doesn't mean that your life has to instantly come to a grinding halt. Every moment that follows your diagnosis will not be terrible; you will still have lots of life to live and lots of joy. You will likely find that you are stronger and more resilient than you thought and that you can continue to lead a high-quality life.

> Let me be clear—I don't subscribe to the view that bad news is a gift. A gift is something gladly given and happily received. Illness is not a gift! Even if illness provides a learning experience, a lesson, an insight, and special memories, illness is not something happily received. To me, that view is Pollyannaish and unrealistic.
>
> I would gladly trade every bit of insight, understanding, wisdom, and act of kindness I gained after my parents' deaths to have them back. Most of my patients wouldn't hesitate to give back all the insights, understanding, wisdom, and acts of kindness they gained during their illnesses for a cure. But if you can gain any good from bad news, any insight from grief—take it!

Yes, things won't be the same; you may have to adapt, adjust, and endure a tremendous amount of loss. Although you'll go through difficult times, not *everything* will be lost, or at least it won't be lost *all at once*. Even if the worst-case scenario occurs, your world won't immediately end.

My dad died suddenly at age fifty-four. It was Valentine's Day. I got a late-night, long-distance call. What a shock. He was way too young. I was crushed and devastated, and I couldn't function. My life came to a halt—but then somehow it went on. And although I miss him terribly, my life has continued, and during that time I've experienced many wonders, numerous blessings, and lots of great joy.

Even if your tomorrows are limited, you can find joy, meaning, and fulfillment today and in the days ahead. You can find appreciation, gratitude, insights, openings, opportunities, and connections. Look for bright spots. At times, they may be hard to see, but they exist. Embrace the goal of living the best you can for as long as you can.

YOUR RESPONSE

When you're diagnosed with a serious illness, be realistic, understand that your life will change. At the same time, be kind and compassionate to yourself, treat yourself well, and enjoy the people and things that make you happy, without feeling guilt or shame.

Tiny pleasures, the small, seemingly minor, things, can help. They can add some luster and enjoyment to your life.

Jim, a spirited but frail seventy-two-year-old, was homebound with advanced heart failure. Although Jim loved his daily scotch, his sons were adamantly against it. They were afraid that if Jim drank even one glass of scotch, it would aggravate his condition, especially since he seemed to be more and more unsteady on his feet. They worried that he might fall. It became a point of contention between Jim and his sons.

When I visited him at home, Jim pulled me aside and asked, "Hey, Doc, would it be OK if I had just one glass of scotch before dinner?" We laughed about how the tables had turned from the time when his sons were in high school and he had admonished them about drinking. Although his sons

strongly objected to Jim drinking *any* scotch, I said, "Sure."
One scotch might have slightly increased his risk of falling,
but it made Jim happy. We talked about limiting it to one
glass a night, and Jim promised to ask for help if he felt unsteady after his nightly drink. With a wry smile, Jim told me
how much he loved that glass of scotch and looked forward
to it. Small as it was, being able to still enjoy it enhanced the
quality of his life.

Late one afternoon before dinner, several months later,
Jim drank what would be his last glass of scotch. After sup-
per, he played poker with his sons and then died peacefully
in his sleep.

Life is how you live; it's what you do. Often, little things
bring great comfort and satisfaction. And you may appreciate
them more. When you're seriously ill, you may cry a lot, but
chances are you will also laugh.

Having a good attitude won't heal you, but it can make a huge
difference. You may feel better if you're proactive and focus on
identifying the best doctors, finding the best treatment and support, and trying to figure out how you can make your situation
better. Being with your favorite people may also help, as can going to your favorite places and doing what you enjoy most—like
drinking a glass of scotch each day.

GRIEF

When we get bad medical news, we grieve; we experience intense
sorrow. The fear and anticipation of loss saddens and upsets us.
When we grieve, we have reactions that were first identified by
the psychiatrist Elisabeth Kübler-Ross and are often referred to
as "stages." These reactions are:

> Denial and isolation
> Anger
> Bargaining
> Depression
> Acceptance

The word "stages" suggests a linear, step-by-step progression starting with denial and isolation and ending with acceptance. For better or worse, the stages of grief are not linear. When we grieve, we don't necessarily experience the five reactions consecutively or in order. We may not go through denial first, then anger, bargaining, and depression before we accept our fate. Acceptance may be fleeting or never come. Grief is not so firmly structured or neat; in fact, it's often chaotic.

It's common for the five reactions to grief to be jumbled, to come at different times and degrees, to come together, to coexist, or to overlap. For example, we may simultaneously be in denial and be angry, or we may be in denial and be depressed at the same time. In quick succession, we may feel anger, bounce to acceptance, and revert to raging anger again.

> When you get bad news, every reaction to grief is normal. Any order, any combination, and any configuration of those reactions are also normal and to be expected. Rather than moving steadily through grief, we may move around it or within it.

When I'm talking with patients, I often hear them express two, or even all, of the stages of grief in a single statement. A patient might say, "Oh, Dr. Pantilat, this is so awful. I feel so low (depression). And it's so unfair; I don't deserve this (anger)! But then, it's really not as bad as they say (denial). Still, I'm going to fight this thing. They said I had six months, but I'm going to fight and live for another ten years (bargaining). But when it's my time, I just want to go peacefully (acceptance)."

It's not unusual to experience multiple stages of grief at the same time, for your emotions to be dizzying and out of control. At one point you may be deeply depressed, and later you may be bargaining. You may say, "If I take these treatments, exercise, and eat right, I'll beat this thing." At other times you may feel overwhelmed and want to give up. And it's also common to go through periods of calm or experience only one reaction at a time.

DENIAL

Denial often gets a bad rap. People tend to equate it with not facing reality. Denial is complex because it can often be helpful. I frequently hear colleagues speak derisively about a patient, saying, "It's so frustrating because he's in denial. He just won't talk about his illness, how serious it is, or the fact that he is dying." Can you blame him?! The poor guy is undergoing toxic chemotherapy. He's weak and thin, his hair has fallen out, he's on a leave of absence from work, and he had to postpone his plans to marry his longtime girlfriend. His silence may be seen as avoidance, at least with respect to some parts of his situation. However, denial may be the only way for him to function and move forward in the face of a string of terrible news and an uphill climb.

If, like the young man I just described, you're making choices that are consistent with your fundamental values, denial may be the best way for you to move forward through your grief, to feel your way, and to do what you need to do to get through the day. It may be the best way for you to diffuse your anguish and pain.

It's essential to distinguish denial from ignoring reality—pretending that nothing is wrong and not moving forward. Turning away, forgetting, or ignoring bad news won't make it go away. In fact, when you ignore bad news, it usually gets worse, much worse than if you had dealt with it right away. That type of denial tends to add layers of trouble, new and unnecessary complications that pile up.

Robert, sixty-two, noticed blood in his stool, which he chalked up to hemorrhoids. He worried that it might be cancer, but quickly dismissed the idea. His bleeding got worse, and he bled daily. After six months, Robert was feeling weak. One morning, he passed out, and he then finally came to the hospital. He told the doctors he thought he had hemorrhoids. Unfortunately, he had colon cancer that had spread to his liver, and his red blood cell count was dangerously low. The oncologist told me that Robert's cancer might have been curable six months earlier, when the bleeding started. Denial was disastrous for Robert.

It's also important to differentiate short-term denial from prolonged denial. Short-term denial can initially help you, but when it's carried too far, it can be harmful and hold you back. Continuous long-term denial can prevent you from taking care of business, doing what's necessary, and doing what's best.

Margaret, a single mother in her early thirties, was slipping fast and didn't have long to live. Although her daughter, Lucy, was only four years old, Margaret had not designated who would raise Lucy in her stead. Somewhere deep down, Margaret may have felt that arranging for Lucy's care would be an acknowledgment of her impending death and an abandonment of hope. However, by not providing for Lucy's care she was ignoring reality. Margaret was not taking care of business—vitally important business.

My team and I had to work through Margaret's denial in order to convince her to do what was most important: provide for Lucy's care. We had to ask the hard questions—questions she was avoiding. We had to find out who Margaret wanted to raise Lucy.

We explained to Margaret that our treatment plan was to give her excellent care and hope for the best. But we also explained that we wanted to help her plan for the worst and do what would be best for Lucy. We stressed that she had to be realistic. Margaret understood, and we helped her put a plan in place. She decided that her mother should raise Lucy. Our social worker helped Margaret talk to her mother and Lucy and arranged for someone to come to the hospital to help Margaret with the necessary legal documents.

Denial can be paralyzing. We recognized that Margaret needed help, and with help, she was able to step out of denial long enough to do what was best for her daughter and herself.

DELIVERING BAD NEWS

It's hard to give bad news. Many doctors don't do it well. Most of us hate giving bad news, especially to patients we like and with whom we've had long relationships. A doctor may have treated a patient for years and worked with him or her to beat some thorny medical problems. Sometimes a doctor has cared for a patient's entire family and has close personal relationships with them. It's easy to understand why doctors may be uncomfortable, nervous, or emotionally upset when we have to deliver bad news. When a doctor delivers bad news, you may notice tears in his or her eyes—after all, we're all just human beings on this journey together.

Regardless of how well doctors deliver bad news, bad news is hard for patients to swallow. It's always unwanted and unwelcomed. I tell my students that bad news—even when delivered as well as possible—is still bad and leaves everyone feeling down. But when the news is delivered with compassion, caring, and empathy, in simple and direct language, by doctors who know when to speak and when to be quiet and listen, it can be easier to take.

Until recently, most doctors weren't taught how to give bad news. Now they are. I teach medical students and doctors to deliver bad news clearly and directly and then be silent. As soon as they give the diagnosis, I suggest that they sit quietly for however long it takes while the patient absorbs the news. I tell them to resist the urge to fill the uncomfortable silence. If we wait calmly, patients usually ask questions and we can respond. After a pause, patients may be better able to understand the additional information we have to give them. If you need time to digest bad news, don't hesitate to ask your doctor to give you a few minutes of silence.

WHY DID THIS HAPPEN TO ME?

When people receive bad news, virtually everyone asks, "Why did this happen to me?" Although no really good answer exists, I say, "It's not fair. Bad things happen, and it's not fair."

Like Richard, people also ask, "Will I die from this?" and "How long do I have?" These questions are natural and totally normal. Many patients also look for something or someone to blame, and many of them blame themselves. I frequently hear them say:

> "I got lung cancer because I smoked."
> "I didn't get a mammogram."
> "I talked too much on my cell phone."
> "I didn't exercise or eat right."
> "I inherited lousy genes."

My response is, "It's still not fair. You didn't choose your parents or to inherit their genes. Even if you smoked, talked endlessly on your cell phone, didn't get a mammogram, didn't exercise, or didn't eat healthy food, it's still not fair! Lots of people do the same and don't get the bad news you just received. It's not fair that this happened to you, and I'm really sorry that it did."

If you believe that you brought this bad news on yourself, that you're to blame, let it go. You don't deserve this bad news, no matter what you may or may not have done. Most serious illness stems from numerous factors, many of which are beyond our control. Your condition may be attributable to traits you were born with or inherited or items that you lived or worked around. Even if you did some things wrong, even many things wrong—as so many of us have—you're probably not the cause of your dilemma. So give yourself a break, don't beat yourself up—have compassion for yourself.

Blaming yourself for something you are or did or didn't do is a waste of time; it doesn't help. It's not fair that you're seriously ill, and placing guilt on yourself won't help. Instead of blaming yourself, have compassion for yourself and see what you can do to move forward.

Even in times of deep despair, anguish, and unfairness, some areas of brightness and hope may exist. Look for them; find them. Instead of blaming and shaming, search for bright spots, things to look forward to and enjoy. Know that what has happened has happened, and it's over. You must move on. Live today—don't relive and regret the past.

RX

At Laguna Honda Hospital, the county-run nursing home in San Francisco, the old hospice unit had a "smoking room" with pictures on the wall of cool people smoking. The idea was that if you were in the hospice unit, dying from an illness related to smoking, it was not the time to add to your feelings of guilt and shame. Since not smoking after you're diagnosed with lung cancer is better for your health and recovery, I encourage and help my patients to quit. However, I appreciated the sentiment behind the "smoking room" and the logic, love, understanding, and compassion it reflected.

Make the most of the time you have because it's precious. It's a gift that not everyone gets. My dad died suddenly at age fifty-four, and I wish we had had the time and opportunity to tell each other one more time what was in our hearts.

chapter two

MOVING FORWARD

AFTER YOU'VE RECEIVED THE BAD NEWS AND YOUR WORST fears have been confirmed:

> Take time to collect yourself.
> Don't make any immediate decisions.
> Sit tight. Let it all sink in.
> Then, when you feel ready, think about your options and how you can move forward.

Moving forward is imperative. Dealing with your illness will give you a mission, a cause that can change your focus. Moving ahead can force you to examine your values and your priorities. Taking the initiative can lift your spirits and inspire you to take action that will help you make the best of your situation. Not moving forward can put you in danger of slipping further into your sorrow and becoming more dejected, even depressed.

Moving forward doesn't always mean immediately beginning aggressive curative treatments. Many people need to start treatment right away, but others don't. All-out assaults may not be called for or what you need or want. You and your medical team should explore how you'll move forward, what's the best course for you. On occasion, it may even be preferable to delay the start of treatments.

When Jack, a patient in his early sixties, was diagnosed with pancreatic cancer, I told him that chemotherapy could help him feel better and might help him live longer, but it wouldn't cure his cancer. As we spoke, I also explained the downsides of chemo, how it could weaken and affect him. Then I asked him what he hoped for, what was important to him, and what he was worried about.

Jack told me that he had been thinking about flying cross-country and visiting his hometown to spend time with his best friend. This trip had been on his mind for a long time, but he hadn't gotten around to it. Now, after getting the diagnosis, it seemed even more important and urgent. Although Jack was eager to start chemotherapy, he was worried that if he did, he might never take this trip.

We spoke with his oncologist, who said that he saw no harm in holding off Jack's chemo for two or three weeks. Jack took a two-week trip to his hometown, and when he returned he began his chemo. Jack's trip buoyed his spirits and gave him a sense of peace that helped him get through his treatments.

Don't assume that treatments will make you feel better, at least not right away. Of course, the hope is that they will, but they may have painful and/or uncomfortable side effects that can prevent you from doing important things such as visiting your hometown or having a big wedding.

Prioritize and realize that while bad news can initially wallop you like a hurricane—and your treatments can feel like another storm, often within the storm or right behind it—you'll find the eye of the hurricane: a place of calm. Embrace these respites. Take advantage of the quiet.

When you think about moving forward, understand that you can't go it alone. Even if you want to, chances are that it won't be possible—you're going to need help. In fact, you may need lots of help. Prepare for it. Don't be proud, reluctant, or ashamed. Let others help you. Don't wait for them to offer—speak up and ask for what you want and need.

Build a support team. Start with those closest to you: people you can rely on, speak with freely and honestly, and vent your feelings to. Then enlist medical professionals: the doctors, nurses, therapists, consultants, and caregivers you're going to need. Add your lawyer, accountant, financial planner, insurance agent, and religious or spiritual advisors—whomever you want or may need.

Try to have everyone on your team in place before you need them. Then, when problems arise, as they inevitably will, you won't have to panic or waste time scrambling for help. You'll know exactly where to turn, whom to call, and what to do. You can move faster and more efficiently if you're prepared.

Those who love you will want to help. Some of them may just show up and ask what they can do, but most will wait to hear how they can help. Tell them.

Create a plan for moving forward. A plan will help you make the most of your time. Don't worry, you don't have to draw up a long, detailed plan; just list some basic points that will get you started. For instance, identify the following:

> The doctor who'll lead your treatment team.
> Whether you'll need specialized care.
> Where you'll get your care. Should you get treatment at a specialized center?
> What information you'll need to learn about your condition and where you can get that information.
> The most important steps to take now.
> What to tell your friends, family, children, and coworkers about your illness.

Since you can't predict the future or know how your condition will progress, your plan will change as you go through it. Most treatment plans do. However, you need to start somewhere, and a basic to-do list will get you focused, organized, and in gear. Then, as you move along, you can make changes and adjustments.

Here's how to begin.

PHYSICIANS

Find a physician to lead your treatment team. Look for someone who will work with you to develop a treatment plan and guide you and your team throughout your illness. Ideally, the physician you choose will understand your condition, know how to treat it, have experience treating it, and help you navigate through it. Find an expert you have confidence in, a doctor who you believe will give you the best information and advice and will work with you to create the best plan.

Start with your personal physician or the doctor who diagnosed your condition. If you have a personal physician you like and trust, you're way ahead of the game. He or she can be your partner throughout your illness. If you don't have a doctor you like and trust, find one.

Will you need a specialist? Your personal doctor may be able to treat common conditions such as straightforward heart disease or lung conditions but may not have the know-how, experience, or expertise to treat more unusual and complex illnesses. Usually, your doctor will tell you if you need a specialist.

For uncommon conditions, your best bet may be to see a specialist in your community. If your condition is rare or highly complex, you may want to go to a specialist at a larger hospital, a specialized medical center, or a university hospital.

Strong evidence shows that patients treated in specialized medical centers by multidisciplinary teams for conditions such as ALS have better outcomes [2.1]. These expert teams have access to the latest research, clinical trials, devices, and equipment. They know the nuances and subtleties of the conditions they treat, so they excel at anticipating issues that might arise and at spotting clues that less experienced clinicians might miss.

In addition to medical treatments, most specialized centers offer a wide range of treatments including medications, physical therapy, exercise, and nutrition. They also have access to and use the latest medical devices and equipment. If you're suffering from a rare or uncommon condition, look into getting treatment at a facility that uses expert, interdisciplinary approaches.

As you look for a physician, keep in mind that physicians differ; they have different personalities, communication skills, and management styles. The key is to find a doctor whose style resonates with you. Some doctors are extremely directive, almost parental, in their approach, which some patients prefer. When you're seriously ill, it's easy to get overwhelmed, and some patients want a doctor who will spell out the course of treatment and tell them exactly what to do. Directive doctors do just that.

Other physicians take a more collaborative approach. They act more like advisors by giving you options and explaining the advantages, disadvantages, time frames, and risks of each course of action. When you work with collaborative doctors, you make the decisions with your doctors' guidance and advice.

Physicians' communication styles and skills also vary. Some can be confusingly technical, even baffling and opaque, while others are crystal clear. Some doctors can be direct, straightforward, and blunt, while others may wander, be indirect, or beat around the bush. Some may come off as all business, impersonal, or cold, while others seem warmer, gentler, and more caring and understanding.

Doctors are human. Most are open, extremely focused, and dedicated to doing the very best for every patient they treat. However, some can be set in their ways and may not listen well or be open to collaborating with you. Find physicians who seem genuinely interested in learning what's unique and special about you and your illness and dedicated to having a partnership with you.

Finding the right doctor, one with a combination of smarts and personality, whose style matches yours, isn't always easy—especially if your illness is rare.

WHAT TO LOOK FOR

When you're looking for a doctor, try to find someone who:

> Has the experience and expertise to give you the best possible medical care; someone who understands your illness and knows what he or she is talking about from a medical standpoint. *First and foremost, look for a doctor who has outstanding medical knowledge and skills.*
> Will listen, not just speak. A doctor who will try to find out what is most important to you, respect your values and beliefs, and help you reach your goals.
> You trust, can talk to, and can confide in, and who will give you answers and information you understand.
> Will be accessible, respond promptly, be patient with you, and give you the time you feel you need.
> Has a manner, style, and approach that feels right for you; a physician who inspires your trust and confidence.
> Has an office and staff that is responsive, easy to work with, and makes you feel welcome and cared for.

Long-term illnesses: If your illness could be lengthy—one that could continue for years or decades—finding the right doctor is extremely important since he or she may end up caring for you for a long time. For patients with conditions that take many years to unfold, factors such as a physician's accessibility, responsiveness, patience, clarity of explanations, and manner take on added significance.

Specialized care: When you need treatment for a rare illness or have to undergo a highly specialized procedure, find the physician with the best technical expertise. In these situations, a specialist's technical expertise is more important than his or her bedside manner. He or she doesn't have to click perfectly with you, because the services provided will be extremely discrete.

Since other doctors will treat you, the specialist who provides only technical procedures doesn't have to become your long-term partner or best friend.

> Getting treatment from a medical specialist far from your home may be too difficult, too inconvenient, too exhausting, or too expensive. However, if you have a rare or complex condition and decide to be treated by your local doctor or a local specialist, consider scheduling at least one consultation with a physician who is an acknowledged expert in treating your condition—even if you have to travel for that appointment.

Often a specialist will reassure you that your local doctor will give you excellent care. He or she can also provide recommendations to you and your local doctor, consult with and advise your local doctor, and tell you know what treatments he or she can offer that your local doctor cannot and what the risks and benefits of those treatments might be. Experts also tend to be more aware of studies and clinical trials you might qualify for.

While a specialist is treating you, your personal physician should continue working with you to make sure that other important medical issues are addressed. Since specialists typically limit their focus to a particular condition such as cancer, heart failure, or dementia, or to specific organs like the liver, lungs, or kidneys, your personal physician should keep track of how your various treatments fit together. He or she can help coordinate the care you receive from different specialists and the medications they prescribe. Your personal physician can help you sift through treatment options and make sure that you reach decisions that are consistent with your values and goals.

> I'm often struck by how little most doctors know about their colleagues. They may know their reputations and may have heard some scuttlebutt at the hospital or through the grapevine, but they usually don't know much about their colleagues' knowledge, technical skill, and manner with patients. Patient A will tell me that a certain doctor I referred him to was really great, but Patient B may say the opposite. Remember that doctors rarely see other doctors interact with patients. What doctors do know is how doctors are with one another. As a result, physicians' recommendations are often based on the fact that they like another doctor and think he is a nice guy, that she's always pleasant and cheerful, that he has published lots of papers, and that he seems competent and has a good reputation.

Nurses, on the other hand, are a terrific source of information about doctors. They work closely with doctors—they're often on the front lines with them—so they know how doctors interact with patients and hospital staff and how well they perform in emergencies. Since nurses assist with procedures, they have excellent insights on doctors' technical skills, dispositions, and bedside manners.

Websites also post opinions about doctors. Like all information on the Internet, proceed with caution! Those who submit comments may have personal agendas or axes to grind. However, when the comments about a doctor are consistent, consider them carefully because they may be insightful and convey important information. Conversely, give isolated and inconsistent comments less weight.

RECOMMENDATIONS

To find the right specialist, start by getting recommendations from your personal physician, other health care practitioners, your friends, and your family. Ask those who give you referrals if they have worked directly with the doctor they recommended and, if so, what their impressions are. Speak with people who have been treated by the physicians recommended. Ask them what they liked, what they didn't like, and if any problems arose. Be specific; try to pin them down.

Asking your doctor and your friends and family for recommendations is a good start. But keep in mind that recommendations are subjective. What makes a great doctor, a great partner, or a great match for one person doesn't necessarily mean that the physician recommended will be right for you. If, however, the same doctor is repeatedly recommended, it's worth checking out that doctor.

INTERVIEWING DOCTORS

For some reason, most people are reluctant to interview doctors or don't think they should. Ironically, they don't hesitate to interview real estate agents, contractors, financial planners, and others before they work with them. They question, compare, and check their backgrounds, experience, and references. But they rarely do the same with doctors—even though the stakes are higher.

Interview doctors before you put your life in their hands—especially when you're embarking on a course of treatment, need a serious operation such as open-heart surgery or a transplant, have a new neurologic disorder, or are diagnosed with cancer.

In some cases, you may not see any reason to interview certain doctors. For example, if you like your cardiologist, why interview other cardiologists when your heart condition gets worse? However, if you're diagnosed with a new and serious illness, such as ALS or colon cancer, you may want to interview several prospective doctors to find the best match.

After you receive bad news, you'll probably have time to interview prospective doctors. Most patients do. During interviews, make sure that everything each doctor tells you is clear and understandable, that you and the physician are on the same page. If the information and impressions you get from different doctors vary, you may want to get other opinions. If, however, all the opinions you get are relatively similar, you'll know that you're on the right track.

Before you interview prospective doctors, do your homework. Look into the doctors' education, qualifications, certifications, specialties, and experience. Check for disciplinary sanctions. This information may be found online. The American Board of Medical Specialties website (www.certificationmatters.org/take -charge-of-your-health-care/check-physician-qualifications.aspx) gives information on doctors' certifications. Consumer Reports (www.consumerreports.org/health/doctors-hospitals/doctor -patient-relationship/check-on-your-doctor.htm) gives information on doctors' qualifications, licensing, patient experiences, and disciplinary actions.

Prepare a list of questions to ask. Use the checklist below as a guide. When you question physicians, make sure that you fully understand their answers, because even when doctors use language we think is simple and clear, we can miscommunicate.

In the ER, I examined Wilma, a thirty-two-year-old woman with asthma. To determine the severity of her condition, I asked her if she had ever been on a breathing machine. "Oh, yes," she said. "Pretty much every time I come to the emergency room, I'm on a breathing machine." By "breathing machine" I had meant a ventilator, a machine about the size of a small microwave oven. A ventilator is connected to a tube that goes into the patient's mouth or nose and down the throat and forces air into the lungs. When people struggle to breathe on their own and could die as a result, they're put on ventilators. Being on a ventilator is memorable, not easily forgotten.

Wilma's reply indicated that she had severe, life-threatening asthma, but when I examined her, I was relieved to find that she didn't seem very sick. However, given her history, I was concerned that her condition could quickly deteriorate, so I immediately ordered a nebulizer, a small, handheld tube that generates a fine mist of medicine that the patient inhales and is then absorbed in the lungs. Nebulizers are fairly standard treatments for asthma in emergency rooms.

After one nebulizer dose, I asked Wilma, "How are you doing?" "Much better, thanks," she replied. "This breathing machine always makes me feel better." I did a double-take. To me the term "breathing machine" meant a ventilator and life-threatening asthma. To Wilma, it was a nebulizer. When I asked a few more questions, I realized that Wilma had never been on a ventilator and her asthma wasn't nearly as severe as I had first thought, which changed the course of treatment I prescribed. I learned a valuable lesson on the importance of communicating clearly.

INTERVIEW CHECKLIST

Before you interview prospective doctors, review the checklist below. Customize the checklist to fit your situation. Make changes to any of the suggested questions and add any questions of your own. During interviews, you or your companion should write down or record the answers you receive, which you can review before making your decision. Here are some questions to ask:

___ Have you treated patients with my condition?

___ If so, approximately how many patients over how many years? (Experience is important, especially for rare conditions, but it should not be your most important consideration because many young, freshly trained doctors are more familiar with the newest treatments than older, more experienced practitioners.)

___ What specific treatments would you recommend for me?

___ What are your treatment objectives for each?

___ What are the advantages and risks of each?

___ How soon will I have to start these treatments?

___ What could happen if I choose not to have these treatments?

___ What other treatments are available to me? (Very important! Your doctor should be able to discuss alternatives with you.)

___ What are the advantages and risks of each of these alternatives?

___ Should I consider any experimental treatments?

___ What are the side effects of the treatments you recommend?

___ How am I likely to feel and for how long?

___ How can I deal with how I will feel?

___ How long will my treatment last?

___ When and how will we know if the treatment is working?

___ What should I expect in the future?

___ If I have questions, how can I reach you?

___ How long will it take to get an answer from you?

___ If issues come up at night or on weekends, how can I get the help I need?

 Experimental treatments are usually not the best first option. In most cases, a proven treatment is the best way to start.

We would all like to have access to *our* doctor 24/7, but that's not realistic. Doctors can't always be available. So most doctors partner with other doctors and share the responsibility to be "on call" after regular office hours. This arrangement gives you access to a doctor at all times, though not necessarily to *your* doctor. For most routine situations, this approach works well, but for serious conditions that entail difficult treatments and side effects, it may be important for you to have access to *your* doctor or to a doctor who (1) works closely with your doctor, (2) knows about you and your condition, and (3) has access to your records.

I usually have a few patients who need to be able to reach me at all times, so I give them my cell phone number. You can ask your doctor for that kind of access, but realize that many doctors are not comfortable with that arrangement, which is not a problem if you have access to another doctor who knows your situation and can promptly respond.

DISSATISFACTION

If, after you start treatment, you don't like or are uncomfortable with your doctor, you have several options:

1. ***Try to fix the problem.*** Discuss the problem with your doctor and try to solve it. For example, you could say,

"When I called and you didn't call me back for three days, I was upset because I needed your help." Most doctors will listen to your concerns and try to fix the problem. But if you don't get the answers you want, switch doctors. After all, it's your life. You have to be absolutely comfortable with your doctors.

2. ***Change doctors.*** If you're dissatisfied with your doctor and don't feel you're getting what you need, try to find a physician you feel better about—even if it's late in your treatment. Continuity is important, but so is fit. Changing doctors every month is a problem, but changing once to find a better match can be a good idea.

3. ***Stick it out.*** Don't switch; remain with the doctor you've known and who knows you, for better or for worse.

I've found that most patients who change doctors don't do it because they're dissatisfied with the quality of the treatments their doctors provide, but because they feel that their doctors are not discussing important issues with them or not acknowledging the severity of their conditions. Essentially, it's a communication problem. When patients feel that they're not improving, many get frustrated. If they feel that their doctors are not leveling with them by acknowledging or addressing reality, they're more likely to consider changing doctors.

INFORMATION

Studies show that information influences patients' decisions. When patients have information, they make different choices than they would have made without that information. Information enables you to be realistic about your illness and treatment options. It helps you understand what could be involved and make the best decisions.

Many doctors don't like to give prognoses to seriously ill patients. They don't really know what will happen and when; they can't predict how long you have or precisely what you might face. However, doctors can make educated guesses. I say more about prognosis in chapter 4.

> Request information; don't wait for it to be offered, because it may not be. Question your doctors regularly. Ask for reports and updates on your condition. Ask about your progress and your prognosis.

Use the Internet wisely. The Internet is now our most popular source of information. As soon as most people get a bad diagnosis, they go online to learn about their illnesses, what they're facing, and what their odds and time frames are. However, all too frequently, patients place too much reliance on what they find on the Internet and don't verify this information with their doctors or other reliable sources.

Be careful! Although the Internet has a wealth of good information, it also has tons that can lead you astray and scare you. Some of that information can be dated or just plain wrong. Sites such as the National Institutes of Health (www.nih.gov), the Mayo Clinic (www.mayoclinic.com), UCSF (www.ucsf.edu), and other university sites tend to be reliable. They contain lots of excellent information that can help you understand more about your illness.

Also be aware that information on the Internet, even postings on the most reliable sites, tends to be generic, whereas the medical information you need to make the best decisions should be specific. Factors such as the exact location, stage, grade, and genetics of a cancer can have crucial effects on treatment regimens, as can the cause, extent, and severity of heart disease. The more you know about your condition, the more specific information on it you can usually find on the Internet. However, what you read may not apply to your situation.

Information you find on the Internet may be vague, oversimplified, or bafflingly complex. It can make things seem a lot better—or much worse—than they actually are. Material on the Internet can toy with your emotions by giving you unrealistic hope or throwing you into a funk. Regardless of what you find, don't let it get you too excited or too discouraged.

On some websites, patients describe their experiences and insights about their illnesses. These sites can provide you with valuable information about treatments, side effects, and support groups. They can help you by making it clear that you're not alone.

That said, personal opinions and observations detailed on Internet sites can also be suspect. Those who post them may shade or distort the truth. They may want to promote the practice of a friend or family member or avenge a grudge. Even when posters' motives are good, their observations and opinions may be based on erroneous assumptions or incomplete information. They may not be objective, insightful, or correct.

Watch out for claims on the Internet that seem too good to be true. They are. Unfortunately, many unscrupulous charlatans work the Internet. They prey on those who are seriously ill. When people are suffering, they can be more vulnerable. They're looking for hope, which can color their thinking. Many become desperate and grasp at straws. Beware of claims, promises, and stories of amazing new breakthroughs and cures. Most are unproven, lack a scientific basis, or are simply bogus.

Since the value of information on the Internet can be questionable, always verify it with your doctor.

Paul, age fifty-three, had a rare, aggressive cancer. Despite multiple cycles of chemotherapy, his disease had spread, and he was hospitalized to help control his pain. Paul had no appetite, had lost weight, and was clearly slipping away. In an effort to help his father, Paul's son combed the Internet and came across a treatment that he hoped would help.

I was at Paul's bedside with his oncologist—an internationally renowned expert in treating this type of rare cancer and someone who is consistently praised by his patients for his compassion and caring—when Paul's son asked him to give Paul the treatment he had found online. Before answering, the oncologist paused. I wondered what he would say. After all, Paul was dying and the oncologist's treatments had not helped.

Then the oncologist said, "No. I'm sorry. I can't give Paul that treatment. As his physician, I have a duty to provide Paul with the best treatments possible." He explained, "In medicine, the best treatments are those that have been tested according to scientific methods. While that doesn't mean there aren't potentially helpful treatments out there, if they're good, they should be rigorously tested before being offered to patients. What I can't risk is giving Paul something that could hurt him. In treating Paul, we'll focus on all the treatments we know will help him feel as good as possible." With that statement, the oncologist reaffirmed his commitment to providing Paul with the best care and not giving him unrealistic hope or potentially harmful or toxic treatments.

That approach now guides me when I confer with my patients.

Again, be cautious with anything you find on the Internet. As a general rule, use material posted on the Internet only as a starting point, as basic information that you can build on and verify. At the very least, *corroborate any information you find on the Internet.* Check it, double-check it, and then check it again with physicians and sources you trust.

> I've never met a physician who didn't want his or her patients to recover. Doctors don't try to hide miracle cures from their patients. They don't reject nontraditional treatments simply because they're inconsistent with their values or what they've been taught. Doctors reject them when they believe there isn't enough hard evidence to definitively show that they work. If we knew that a certain herb would cure cancer, we would unhesitatingly prescribe it to all our cancer patients. We might even grow it ourselves!
>
> Before buying or taking an expensive miracle cure (somehow they all turn out to be expensive), demand proof that they've been tested according to scientific methods and that they really work—especially those that have side effects, entail risks, and are costly. We all wish that the miracles promised on the Internet and by far-off clinics worked. Sadly, they don't. And in pursuing them, we often lose precious time and fail to focus on more important care.

INTEGRATIVE MEDICINE

Today, a huge variety of medical treatments are available. Some are nontraditional, and the benefits of many are unproven. Nontraditional practices are frequently referred to as alternative medicine or alternative medical practices. I prefer to refer to them as integrative medical practices in order to reflect that these treatments are integrated into overall, holistic treatment plans. While I'm not an expert on these treatments, I fully support integrative medical practices for serious illness when (1) they have been fully tested and (2) they're part of and complement an overall treatment plan that includes mainstream medical treatments.

Acupuncture, meditation, massage, healing touch, and yoga are some of the most popular integrative practices, but the term also includes other therapies. Not only have many integrative practices been proven to be beneficial, but none have been shown to pose harm, especially when performed by trained practitioners. And these treatments help many people feel better.

The danger with integrative approaches comes when you think of them as cures, not simply as adjuncts to your overall medical treatment. **Warning:** With integrative approaches, trust well-trained medical practitioners who make reasonable assertions on how they can help. Be wary of those with questionable credentials and those who promise cures that seem miraculous.

PALLIATIVE CARE

Now I would like to introduce you to a relatively new medical field that has been proven to be extremely helpful to people with serious illness—palliative care. Unfortunately, few people know about palliative care and many of them misunderstand it. I'm passionate about palliative care. It's my specialty and I've seen how much it helps. Later in this book, I devote an entire chapter to palliative care (chapter 12), but for now I want to highlight a few important points.

Palliative care helps seriously ill patients have *the best possible quality of life* during the course of their curative medical treatments. When given along with treatment for their illnesses, palliative care helps patients live better and longer [2.2]. Palliative care also helps patients' families and friends weather their loved ones' ordeals.

Traditionally, Western medicine deals with patients' illnesses and diseases by trying to eliminate them. However, some diseases cannot be eliminated, and some treatments are harsh, even toxic. They can cause great pain and discomfort, be disabling, and put patients' lives on hold. In trying to eradicate an illness, traditional treatments often do more harm than good, especially late in an illness. Palliative care, which is given along with standard medical treatments, provides an extra layer of support that helps patients function better, be more comfortable, and experience less pain and stress.

Palliative care goes beyond most traditional medical approaches because it's based on the belief that serious illness isn't purely biological. It reflects the realization that serious illness involves numerous factors, including pain, stress, emotions, spiritual beliefs, culture, finances, nature, and values. Palliative care focuses on the *whole person* as well as on his or her particular illness and recognizes that each patient and each illness is unique. As a result, palliative care specialists explore each patient's wants, needs, feelings, background, experiences, and attitude. Then they consider the impact of the illness on each patient medically, emotionally, psychologically, and spiritually and customize a course of treatment for each patient.

BE OPEN AND SPEAK UP

Don't hide your diagnosis. Tell your close friends and family. Although your illness may be hard for you to talk about, remaining silent will isolate you from the help and support you will need. Plus, you'll probably feel better when you speak up. Remember that those who care about you will want to help, but they can't help if they don't know that you're ill. And don't worry that they may feel that you're burdening or imposing on them—they won't.

Before we go any further, I want to acknowledge that I understand that we live in a diverse, multicultural society where people deal with illness, treatment, and communication differently and often in their own traditional ways. When medical problems arise, family members may try to protect their loved ones and demonstrate their concern by following their cultural traditions, which may include shielding their loved ones from the truth. Since this issue is common, complex, and nuanced, I discuss it and its effect in detail, in chapter 14.

When you tell others about your illness:

› Be straightforward and direct.
› Explain what you're dealing with, the impact of your illness, and how you feel.
› Keep it simple and don't bore them with all the gory details.

Be open to questions and try to answer them honestly and clearly without going into too much medical or technical detail. Although it's important to tell people about your illness, don't feel compelled to tell everyone everything or to tell it to them all at once. Some things are private, and the timing may not be right. Share only what you feel comfortable with and remember that you don't have an obligation to reveal everything to everyone.

When you tell others, be prepared for a variety of responses. Many people will be supportive. They'll listen with interest and empathy and keep the focus on you. Others will want to share their medical stories with you. They may identify with you and your story and want to bond over the news. Or they may simply need to discuss their own experience. Sometimes their stories will be helpful. They can put your situation in perspective, provide insights, and give you support and strength. But sadly, all too frequently, other people's personal stories are off-base and off-putting.

When people share personal stories that don't seem helpful, feel free to interrupt or cut them off. Explain that right now, given your situation, it's hard for you to hear about other people's experiences. Those who really care about you will understand.

People can be insensitive. Most don't intend to be hurtful, but they can be. Frequently, when they learn that others are seriously ill, they try to distinguish themselves. They try to convince themselves that they're different and, therefore, not likely to get the same illness or disease. The most common example is asking someone with lung cancer, "Did you smoke?"

Avoid these types of questions. They rarely serve any useful purpose because we all differ, as do the reasons for our illnesses. Plus, these self-serving questions usually make those who are already suffering feel worse.

The plain truth is that serious illness is sad, and we don't want to make it worse. Most seriously ill people are reeling, and you can bet that a smoker who has lung cancer has already beaten him- or herself up for it—over and over again. Furthermore, the question can be painful for nonsmokers because it magnifies the unfairness of their situation at a time when they're still struggling with their bad news. Better to say, "I'm so sorry. How are you doing?"

SUPPORT

When you learn that you're seriously ill, you have many needs. Perhaps the most pressing is the need for moral and emotional support. When you receive a bad diagnosis, talk to people who know you, love you, and care about you. Although they won't be able to fix your problem or make it go away, they can be with you, stand by you, root for you, and listen to you with compassion, empathy, patience, and concern. Their support can give you strength as you move forward.

Some folks are ashamed or embarrassed that they're ill. They keep to themselves and don't reach out. Don't fall into that trap. *When you're seriously ill, it's not the time for isolation. It's time to marshal support and rally the troops.* Serious illness is not a moral failing; it's a life-changing event that's not your fault. You may not want to advertise your bad news or post it on the Internet, but reach out, get help and support!

> Don't try to be heroic and don't stand alone. Let people who care about you lighten your load. Their help will make the journey easier, better, and more meaningful for you and your loved ones. Many people will volunteer to help. Let them.

Your friends and family can help with your practical needs, or they can simply keep you company. They can give you rides to medical appointments, run errands, make phone calls, shop, clean, and take care of other chores and business. They can lessen your burdens so you can focus your time and energy on your health.

When Kathy was going through chemotherapy for breast cancer, she lost her hair. Losing her hair made her feel so self-conscious that she kept to herself and hardly left home. One day, my friend Susan showed up at Kathy's house and told her that they were going wig shopping. Susan, who had done her research, took Kathy to a great place. Kathy chose a new wig, put it on, and they went to lunch.

Their outing really lifted Kathy's spirits. She didn't feel self-conscious—in fact, she thought she looked good. She needed a wig, but she didn't want to go shopping alone. Plus, she was too embarrassed to ask for help. Somehow, Susan understood Kathy's feelings and knew the difference between just offering help and actually giving it.

Some people will disappear. They might find your illness threatening or frightening. It may raise issues about their own mortality or remind them of other painful losses they suffered. They may be too sad or worried to reach out to you. Or it may simply be a bad time for them.

People will stay away because they're afraid that they won't know what to say or will say or do something wrong. When you find that those you thought you could rely on have disappeared, let them know that you would like their help. Don't scold or chastise them. Simply tell them not to be frightened or embarrassed. Reassure them that it's OK for them to say nothing and just be with you. Explain that their companionship, friendship, and caring is important to you and that's what you need most. When you don't know what to say, just speak from the heart.

On the other hand, some well-meaning individuals will get in the way. They truly want to help but end up doing the opposite.

Try giving them jobs that will keep them out of the way. Assign them basic, uncomplicated tasks such as running errands or making calls—jobs they can't mess up—and give them precise instructions. If they still get in the way, explain that you know that they mean well and that you appreciate their efforts, but they're complicating matters and making it more difficult for you. Or you might say, "Thank you. Right now I have all the help I need. If I need you or have questions, I will be in touch."

The fact that you're ill doesn't mean that you have to accept the company of everyone who offers it or talk about your illness all the time. Tell your family and friends how you feel. When you don't want to talk about your illness, say so and change the subject. Understand that your feelings may fluctuate. At times, you may want to discuss your illness, your mortality, and your grief, and at other times, you may not.

Frequently, those who are ill won't ask for help because they don't want to be a burden to others. However, their friends and family don't look at it that way. They consider helping to be a blessing and a privilege.

At a conference on how to communicate with sick patients, I took part in a role-playing exercise. I played the part of a patient who had advanced cancer and was worried that he had become a burden to his wife. I was instructed to act sad and ashamed. I expressed those feelings to Dr. Ira Byock, a friend and a wonderful palliative care physician, who was playing my doctor. Ira asked me, "If your wife was in your situation, would you consider it a burden to care for her?"

Even though we were acting, my eyes welled up with tears. "Of course not," I immediately replied, and I meant it.

"If caring for your wife, whom you love so much, would not be a burden for you," Ira said, "why would you think that your wife, who loves you, would feel differently?"

> If you have a friend or family member who is seriously
> ill, be a friend—help. Don't wait to be asked. Bring
> dinner. Buy groceries. Do laundry. Take the kids for the
> day or for a few hours. Instead of just asking what you
> can do, find ways to help.

Your coworkers also care about you. Talk with your colleagues
to fill them in on your situation. You may need to take time off
and may feel guilty about saddling others with more work. Knowing what you're going through will help both you and your coworkers. They can plan for your absences, make adjustments,
hire temporary help, place projects on hold, or shift assignments
and tasks. When you have to miss work, they may want to visit
you, help you, and be part of your team.

WHAT TO TELL THE KIDS

If you have children or grandchildren in your life, you may wonder what to tell them. If your illness isn't obvious, won't be obvious for some time, and isn't likely to suddenly get worse, it may
be best to say nothing at this time. No need to scare children
unnecessarily and make them worry.

However, hiding a serious illness may not be possible if it
causes major life changes, has serious, noticeable side effects, or
involves hospitalization. Kids can also be sensitive and intuitive.
Despite your smiles, cheerfulness, and reassurances, they may
detect that something is amiss. They may hold it in, worry, and
suffer silently. So watch for behavioral regression, emotional outbursts, and the need for increased attention, which are clues to
how they're actually feeling. These behaviors are signs that you
need to discuss the illness with your children.

When and what to tell kids will differ according to the circumstances, the children, their ages, and their sensitivities. Usually, the older the child, the better he or she will understand and
the more you may want to disclose.

Above all else, children need reassurance. A simple explanation that you're sick and getting treatment may be enough. Tell
your child or grandchild the name of your illness—for example,
"cancer" or "emphysema." Naming the illness will help make the
illness seem like a distinct and separate entity from yourself. Explain that you are seeing doctors who are working with you to
help you feel better. Answer questions directly and simply. As a
rule of thumb, I suggest that you just answer the question you're
asked. Here is a brief example:

"What's wrong?"

"Mommy is sick and not feeling well, but I'm getting help
from the doctor to feel better."

"Will you get better?"

"I plan on it!"

It is very important to reassure young children that your
illness is not their fault, as children are egocentric and tend to
blame themselves for disruptions in the family. Explain that illness just happens to people, and it is never a child's fault. Reassure them that you love them and are doing all you can to feel
better. *A Tiny Boat at Sea* by Izetta Smith (Grief Watch, 2nd edition, 2000) is a wonderful book on talking with young children
about a parent with cancer.

In chapter 14, I go into greater detail on what to say to children, including what to tell them when the news gets worse and
how to answer the hard questions.

RX

Serious illnesses progress at different rates. Some move so quickly that you feel you're out of control. You can barely catch your breath. It's all hurry up—get treatment—make decisions now—change your life today. You're constantly besieged by new problems that demand more urgent action. You feel like you're in a storm or falling off a cliff. That's how it felt for us with my mom's lung cancer. We felt like we were barreling down a mountain and unable to stop.

For most people, serious illness unfolds over a period of many months, even years. If you have time, pace yourself. Put good systems in place; build a great team. Take time to find doctors you trust and feel comfortable with. Enlist friends to help and be with you. If your treatment can wait a bit, think about taking advantage of the calm before the treatment storm.

chapter three

MAKING DECISIONS: HIDDEN FACTORS

DURING YOUR ILLNESS, YOU'LL HAVE TO MAKE MANY DE-cisions. Some of those decisions will be easy, no-brainers that you can immediately make. Others will be difficult, complex, and even baffling. Many of those decisions will be important, and the stakes will be high. At times, you'll feel as if you have no good choices, only bad ones. Still, you need to decide, because not doing so is choosing the status quo.

To make the best decisions, create a two-pronged plan. In prong one, identify your overall goal, what you hope for. In prong two, develop the plan to get you there.

PRONG ONE

Your overall goal may be to wipe out your cancer, to eliminate all traces of it. Or it could be to regain the lost functions caused by your stroke, to get back to work, to travel, to slow your Alzheimer's, or to spend time with loved ones. The goal you set will be the guiding light for your treatment.

Base your goal on your priorities—what's most important to you. Talk with those you can rely on and trust. Get their input. Consider all the opinions you get. Take your time, if you can. Think your decision through. As you do, listen to your emotions, your innermost feelings, how you instinctively feel. Don't dismiss those feelings if they seem irrational or overly emotional, or if they conflict with accepted wisdom, because they reflect the sum total of your experience, your essence, your nature, and who you truly are. Bear with me as I keep emphasizing the importance of identifying your goals and understanding the potential risks and benefits of treatments. They're the essential issues in making treatment decisions. Know your goal. Only then can you use the information you get on the risks and benefits to decide whether a treatment is worth the risk (explored further in chapter 10).

Think about traditional beliefs, the values that have been drummed into you since birth. Are they still relevant to you? Do they reflect how you actually feel, or are they the views of others? You may be surprised how your values have changed over time and how they've been affected by your illness. Is fighting your illness no matter what still critically important to you? Are you worried that someone will see you as a quitter? How do you define quality of life?

For many people, living longer is all that matters, and they can't consider anything else. They will endure torturous pain and spend fortunes in order to prolong their lives. Living longer can have tradeoffs. Longer may not be longer in your home, may not be breathing on your own, and may not be being able to eat, walk, talk, and/or sleep. Fighting can divert, deplete, or exhaust your resources and prolong a battle you can't win. Treatments that you think will help you live longer may fail and instead shorten your life or lessen its quality.

While you're working to set your goal, educate yourself. When it comes to education, I've found that people fall into two groups: (1) those who want all the information they can get and (2) those who only want the bare minimum. The people in group 1 will work hard and read everything they can get their hands on. They will sift through medical journals, spend hours on the Internet, and consult with lots of doctors. They'll also read textbooks and reach out to anyone they think might help. In contrast, those in group 2 won't read; they won't ask scores of questions. All they want is the bottom line, and they'll accept what they're told. They don't want all the details.

If you belong in group 1, start by reading. Learn about your illness and what it entails. Speak with doctors who specialize in your illness and talk to people who also suffer from it. Ask them about their experiences and get their advice. You can find information posted by people with similar illnesses on hospital websites and on sites such as Patients Like Me (www.patientslikeme.com). Also check with organizations that focus on specific conditions, such as the American Cancer Society (www.cancer.org), American Heart Association (www.heart.org), American Lung Association (www.lung.org), Alzheimer's Association (www.alz.org), and others. Sites for hospitals, medical centers, and medical schools provide a wide range of valuable medical information. I especially like UCSF (www.ucsfhealth.org/patients/), the Mayo Clinic (www.mayoclinic.org), and Johns Hopkins Medicine (www.hopkinsmedicine.org/healthlibrary/conditions/adult/).

Learn about your options and what treatments may be available for you. Discover the advantages and disadvantages of each and pay special attention to those that feel right for you. As I mentioned in chapter 2, be cautious about what you read on the Internet. Corroborate it carefully.

If you're in group 2 and want just enough information, meet with a doctor you trust. Think about getting a second opinion. For major treatments like bone marrow transplants or major surgery, you might want to talk to someone who has gone through those treatments. Remember that you're likely to talk to someone who got through treatment well. Even so, their experience may be helpful.

As you're identifying your priorities and goals, examine whether they're feasible. Ask yourself:

> › Can they be achieved?
> › If so, at what cost?
> › What support will I need?
> › Who will provide the support I need?
> › Can I go it alone?

PRONG TWO

How do you hope to reach your goal? In prong two, list the steps you'll take. These steps don't have to be precise or exhaustively detailed. Feel free to start with a loose outline and fill in the gaps as you go along. During your illness, the steps in your plan will change—the best-laid plans for getting through serious illnesses invariably do. But you have to start somewhere, and the best starting point is to make a plan. Creating a plan:

> › Helps you focus on how you're going to get through your illness.
> › Forces you to be proactive—to learn, think, and act to help yourself.

> › Helps you talk to and understand your doctors and other caregivers.
> › Gives you a mission that can help you throw off the funk that's gripped you since you got your bad news.

Examine your treatment options. For each option ask yourself, "Will this treatment help me reach my goal?" Is surgery right for me? What about radiation? Or dialysis?

In some situations, you may need to immediately spring into action and undergo invasive or aggressive treatments. In others, you may be able to take your time to consider options—for example, whether you're willing to have dialysis or to get a left ventricular assist device (LVAD) implanted for your heart failure.

Severe conditions may require serious treatment. You may have to act fast. You also may be faced with an agonizing choice or be forced to conduct a seemingly impossible balancing act—death in days or weeks without treatment versus the risk of death from the treatment. Bone marrow transplants for acute leukemia are an example of this dilemma.

Sometimes the best treatment for you is obvious. At other times, you'll have options, and which path is best may not be clear. Each may have varying degrees of pluses and minuses, so you'll have to compare and contrast to decide what you want to do. Or you may mix and match: go for parts of different types of treatments.

Remember, you have options, including the option not to take treatments for your illness. For example, if you've been diagnosed with incurable cancer, you can decide not to have chemo. You can say no thank you.

My mother-in-law, Shirley, was a whip-smart free spirit who made her own decisions. When she developed abdominal pain and a CT scan showed that she had a mass in her pelvis, she found a surgeon she trusted to remove it to relieve her pain. The surgery helped the pain, but it also revealed that she had fallopian tube cancer. The surgeon referred her to an oncologist who outlined a chemotherapy plan. Shirley listened, asked a lot of questions, and never went back. She weighed the options and decided that the chemotherapy was not worth it. It would make her feel too sick too often for the small chance that she would feel better or live longer.

Shirley outlived her prognosis by a year and credited forgoing chemotherapy with keeping her healthier longer. Although chemotherapy was not the right choice for Shirley, it could be for other patients with cancer. So I'm not suggesting that everyone make the same decision, but I do want to make it clear that you have choices—including the choice not to undergo disease-focused treatments.

A study published in 2015 by my friend Holly Prigerson and her colleagues titled "Chemotherapy Use, Performance Status, and Quality of Life at the End of Life" [3.1] examined the effect of chemotherapy in people who had advanced, incurable cancer. Keep in mind that chemotherapy is given to patients with incurable (metastatic) cancer in order to help them live longer and have a better quality of life. It's not given to make the cancer go away, because at that stage, it can't. The study followed the participants and compared how those who chose chemotherapy and those who did not fared. The researchers grouped the participants into three groups: (1) those who had a good quality of life at the outset of the study, (2) those who had a moderate quality of life, and (3) those who reported that their quality of life was poor. The study followed the participants until they died and then surveyed their loved ones to understand the participants' quality of life near the end of their lives.

What the study found should make us all take pause:

> Chemotherapy had no effect on how long participants lived. Those who chose chemotherapy did not live longer.
> Chemotherapy did not improve the participants' quality of life. In fact, those who had the best quality of life at the outset of the study were also the most likely to get chemotherapy, and the chemotherapy diminished their quality of life.

Sometimes less is more.

One caveat: This study was completed in 2008, and medicine has continued to advance. New treatments are being introduced all the time, and hopefully some will be game changers. With new or current treatments, you must continually remind yourself of your goal and ask, "Will this treatment make it more likely that I achieve it?"

When doctors and patients talk about treatments, they tend to discuss them in terms of their "success." But what does that mean? Whether a treatment is successful depends entirely on how you define success. Think of success in terms of whether a treatment helps you achieve your goal. I've known of treatments that have been called successful because they shrank cancers or eliminated infections, but they also made the patient miserable. The treatments not only failed to help those patients reach their goals; they also made achieving these goals impossible.

THINKING ABOUT TREATMENTS

Treatments themselves are neither good or bad, right or wrong, helpful or harmful. All treatments have risks, and their benefits are never guaranteed. Whether they're right for you depends on if they'll help you achieve your overall goal.

During the course of your treatment, your options and goals can change. Prepare to be flexible so you can quickly move in new directions when it seems best to do so.

Mary was a seventy-six-year-old woman with colon cancer that had spread throughout her abdomen and to her lungs. Her cancer caused fluid to fill her abdomen at an alarming pace. The fluid created intense pressure and caused Mary great pain. Fortunately, we were able to do a "tap"—to place a needle in Mary's abdomen to remove some fluid—and it gave her relief. Unfortunately, the fluid would re-accumulate within a day, so we had to drain it most days.

When I met with Mary and asked her what her goal was, she said, "To get a Denver shunt." A Denver shunt is a plastic tube placed under the skin with one end in the abdomen and the other in a large vein in the neck. The pressure of the fluid in the abdomen pushes it through the tube and into the blood stream. Inserting a Denver shunt was a risky procedure for someone who was as sick as Mary. It tends to have complications and over time stops working. But it was offered as an option, and Mary wanted it.

We took a step back and asked Mary, "When you look to the future, what do you hope for?" "I want to go home, to be able to go out to dinner and visit my grandchildren," she said. "The pain from the fluid in my abdomen and the frequent taps are making that impossible." With Mary's goals in mind, we consulted a liver specialist, who recommended a simpler and safer procedure: placing a tube directly into Mary's abdomen with a valve that she could turn on and off. That way she could drain the fluid whenever it made her uncomfortable.

The Denver shunt was not the real goal; it was a means, and not the right one. With the end goal clear, we could figure out the best means.

> Know your goal. Research all possible treatments. Learn the benefits and drawbacks of each treatment and evaluate the likelihood that it will help you reach your goal.
>
> When you create your plan, remember that life is like an airplane flight. A flight can't take off until a flight plan is filed that shows the destination and the route the flight will take. Ideally, that plan will be direct and avoid all other air traffic and turbulent weather. If all goes as planned, you should enjoy a safe, comfortable ride. Your plan for dealing with your illness can also help you get a smooth, comfortable ride and respond to the inevitable bumps that arise.

Sadly, many people undergo treatments and continue to suffer. They don't get better. They live longer, but they and their loved ones pay a steep, agonizing price.

Multiple heart attacks had left Jim, a seventy-year-old man, with a heart so scarred that it could barely pump. Just walking from room to room at home made him short of breath and brought on chest pain. His legs were horribly swollen, and medications couldn't reduce the swelling. If Jim drank a bit too much water, he would end up in the hospital, short of breath and needing intravenous medications to get him through. We knew that, before long, he wouldn't make it because his heart was so weak that our medicines would fail.

Jim was realistic about his condition and asked if anything could give him relief. His cardiologist talked to him about a left ventricular assist device (LVAD), a pump that is surgically implanted in the chest and connected to the heart to help pump blood. The LVAD has cables that run out of the body and connect to a battery. Although LVADs can be life-saving, they can also cause bleeding, strokes, and infections. Nevertheless, Jim wanted it.

Unfortunately, nothing went right after Jim's surgery. He was never able to breathe on his own, remained sedated on a ventilator, and suffered one complication after another. After three months of hoping that we could overcome the complications, we again met with his daughter, whom Jim had designated as his decision maker. We asked her again what her father's goals were and what he would tell us to do if he could see himself in this situation. His daughter said that her dad's goal was to ride a motorcycle. It was his passion, and heart disease had taken it from him. It was clear that Jim would never have the chance to ride a motorcycle. People with LVADs can't ride motorcycles, ever. I couldn't help but think that we could have figured out how to get him a ride before the LVAD. Of course, hindsight is 20/20, but Jim's goal was clear, and the treatment—even if it had been wildly successful—would not have gotten him any closer to it.

How much are you willing or able to take on or put yourself and your loved ones through? Are you willing to take on harsh, uncomfortable treatments to try to wipe out your illness, or do you want to take a more gentle approach that will be less physically and/or mentally taxing? Are you willing to go to the ICU and be hooked up to ventilators and machines? Or do you want to remain at home?

TREATMENT DECISIONS

In most cases, different types of treatments are available. Your doctors will outline your options. Some doctors will simply give you information about what may be involved and leave the decisions up to you. Others will offer their opinions. In addition, you'll probably hear or read about other approaches that you can ask your doctors about.

The best decisions are informed decisions, so learn about your illness, your prognosis, the treatment options, and what may be involved. Treatments including surgery, chemotherapy, radiation, transplants, implants, and medications often involve hidden factors that you probably don't know about or that health care providers may not have adequately discussed with you.

My friend and colleague Dr. Toby Campbell, who directs the Palliative Care Program at the University of Wisconsin–Madison, along with colleagues has developed a "Best Case/Worst Case" approach that enables doctors to give patients information in a way that helps them make the best treatment decisions. The method works best when patients have a distinct choice— for example, surgery or no surgery for lung cancer, or starting dialysis or not for kidney failure. Toby teaches doctors to answer three questions: (1) what the best and worst outcomes would be as a result of a treatment, (2) what the best and worst outcomes would be without the treatment, and (3) the likely outcome for each. In some situations, even the best outcome with treatment may not be good enough. Or the outcome without treatment could be so good that undergoing treatment would seem like a bad idea. But in other situations, the high likelihood that treatment would provide a good outcome would make the patient's decision obvious.

Toby's tool can help in all treatment decisions that require patients to choose between two options. If you have to make this type of decision, ask your doctor these Best Case/Worst Case questions. Your doctor's answers can help you decide which treatment is best for you.

To help you make the best, most enlightened decisions, some of the more common treatments are listed later in this chapter, with information on hidden factors that could be involved with each.

When you make treatment decisions, keep in mind the following:

> When doctors estimate the odds of recovery, they're making "educated" guesses based on their experience—but they're still guesses. When they tell a patient that surgery has a 50 percent chance of providing relief, they can't predict the results for that patient. They also don't know what they're going to find when they operate. It could be what they expect or worse.

> Not fighting as hard as you can is not giving up. Neither is refusing to undergo aggressive, invasive, or harsh treatments. And fighting as hard as you can is not always the approach that will provide the best outcome. It's complex. Treatments that have worked for others may not be right for you. The bottom line is that the treatments you undergo must be right for you. The question that must be answered is, "How likely are you to get the benefits that usually come from those treatments? Will those treatments get you to your goal?" Again, get information and listen to your gut. Be true to yourself.

> In reflective, private moments, many patients have admitted to me that they didn't want a certain treatment, but they agreed to it because their loved ones desperately wanted them to or because they didn't want to be seen as quitters. Whenever I hear this, I want to cry. Often, these patients have been through hell, and the thought of considering them anything but brave is a joke. My mother-in-law, Shirley, who refused chemotherapy, was not a quitter. She fought hard to live and live well, but without chemo.
>
> As hard as it is to think about losing someone you love, I can't imagine any loved one wanting someone they care about to undergo treatment they don't want simply to appease others. Although friends and family are well-intentioned, they frequently don't understand how particular treatments could affect your quality of life or your ability to be with loved ones, stay out of hospitals, and do what you enjoy.

› Treatments have three possible outcomes: they can make your condition better, keep it the same, or make it worse. Virtually all treatments have side effects and produce new issues that must subsequently be addressed. Side effects can slow or impede recovery or even outweigh the benefits of treatments. Family and friends frequently don't know or understand the hidden factors, risks, and side effects. In their desire to see you recover, they may pressure you to make decisions that don't sit well with you.

› Ask, "Will the results apply to me?" Many patients base their treatment decisions on the findings of clinical studies, which is reasonable and understandable. However, too often people who would have been excluded from studies because they were too sick assume that the study findings would apply to them. Be especially cautious about applying the findings of clinical studies to those who would have been excluded from the studies.

Treatments studied do not benefit every patient who participates in the study; they never do. Nothing in medicine is 100 percent, and we don't expect it to be. Although the treatment helped some patients, it may not help you. Your case may differ from those studied because of your age, health, genetics, medical history, lifestyle, and tolerances.

Patients frequently misunderstand clinical trials, especially Phase I clinical trials. Clinical trials are experiments designed to see if treatments work. We only study treatments when we don't know whether they're effective. Phase I clinical trials are a special category: they're toxicity tests. They test only whether a treatment is toxic, not whether the treatment is curative. Even though patients are explicitly told that a Phase I trial will not examine therapeutic benefits, people assume that we wouldn't study treatments if we didn't think that they would help.

> When my patients are considering enrolling in a clinical trial, I tell them that the reason to enroll is to advance science, not to find a cure for their illness. I applaud them and am grateful for their participation. Most of the treatments we have today are available because people courageously and altruistically enrolled in a clinical trial. However, we also need to remember that many treatments tested in clinical trials don't pan out, many are not quite as good as hoped, and a few are downright harmful.

> People tend to believe that the odds will be in their favor. When they're told that a certain treatment has been shown to have a 30 percent success rate, they're convinced that they'll be in that 30 percent. I don't blame them. When you agree to any treatment, you have to believe that it will work. Not only that, you must believe that you'll sail through and have no horrible side effects. Since both doctors and patients hope for the best, they often avoid asking the hard questions. Doctors, in their desire to help, and patients, in their hope for a cure, don't always realistically look at each situation—a failing that can make bad situations worse.

> Treatments fall into two categories: those that can be stopped and those that cannot. Dialysis can be stopped at any point. Patients who have kidney failure undergo dialysis because they would die without it. However, dialysis does not improve the ability to function or the quality of life of patients with advanced diseases like dementia. In fact, dialysis can make their condition worse [3.2]. So can giving them artificial nutrition via feeding tubes, or antibiotics. Major surgery, implanting pumps for failing hearts, and bone marrow transplants can't be undone. Once you commit to undergoing these treatments, you take on both the possible benefits and the risks. Surgery may require significant recovery and healing, and transplants are permanent. Ask your doctor whether recommended treatments are reversible or permanent. Think long and hard before agreeing to those that are permanent. Remember, you always have options.

A tension exists between the two common sayings "No risk, no reward" and "What have I got to lose?" Many serious illnesses require risky treatments, and I believe in medicine and the power of treatments to help people feel better. I've seen remarkable recoveries. Some risk is inevitable when you decide to undergo treatment. And some treatments expose you to great risk, but they may provide great rewards. However, I worry when I hear, "Hey, what have I got to lose? If the treatments don't work, at least I tried something that might have worked."

Only undergo a treatment if it has a reasonable chance of succeeding, not because it's simply something to try. You could lose a lot—your strength, your time—and suffer the fallout from devastating complications. The sicker you are, the greater the odds are against you. If you're fragile, your condition is more likely to get worse. Accept risk, but only when you also have the realistic possibility of benefit.

Like life, medicine is lived in real time and is inherently uncertain. When you have to make a major treatment decision, ask a lot of questions, gather the best evidence, make an informed decision, and then don't look back. Don't drive yourself crazy rethinking your decisions. The decision you made probably was the best one you could have made at the time. If it didn't work out as you had hoped, it doesn't mean that your decision was incorrect; your disease may have been too powerful for the treatments, or you could have just been unlucky.

When Carol was seventy-eight, she was diagnosed with pancreatic cancer. At the time, she was living at home with her husband, walking every day, and traveling. The diagnosis came as a huge surprise, as it so often does, and unfortunately her cancer had already spread at the time of her diagnosis. Pancreatic cancer tends to be found in a more advanced state because it doesn't cause much in the way of symptoms until late in its progression. It also doesn't respond well to chemotherapy.

After the initial shock, Carol was hell-bent on getting treatment as soon as possible. The thought that the cancer was growing inside her made her crazy. The next day, she saw an oncologist and immediately began chemotherapy. The chemotherapy made her so sick that she refused the second dose. Over the next few months, Carol's condition deteriorated, she lost a lot of weight, had no appetite, and was too weak to leave her home.

When I visited her at home, she asked if I thought the chemotherapy had caused her to feel so sick so quickly. I told her, "No." She asked if stopping chemotherapy let the disease progress quickly and if she should have taken more chemo. Again, I said, "No." I explained that it wasn't fair that she had gotten so sick so quickly. That when cancer has progressed so rapidly, chemotherapy isn't likely to help and may have made her feel worse. I reassured her that she had made good decisions—to try chemo and then to stop when it made her sick. Her decisions were extremely reasonable at the time.

It's not fair that you got cancer or heart failure or any other serious illness, and it's also not fair that your illness would gallop along so quickly. So don't beat yourself up for doing your best, for trying to make the best decisions at the time. Don't add to the challenges you face. Be kind to yourself. Practice self-compassion. Look forward to the life you still have to live, not backwards to the past, which you cannot change.

HIDDEN EFFECTS

Not everyone responds well to surgery, radiation therapy, or other aggressive techniques. Often patients' response, or lack of it, is caused by hidden factors that they didn't know about or consider sufficiently. Be realistic about the treatments you're considering. Find out how they can both help and hurt.

The following are some hidden effects you may not be aware of:

Surgery: After surgery, you'll have a wound that has to heal. As it does, you'll also have short-term pain from your operation. Your recovery will usually depend on the extent of your operation and how sick you were going in. However, exceptions always occur. I've seen patients who were dying from advanced liver disease make remarkable recoveries just days after liver transplants, which are among the most major operations you can undergo. Unfortunately, I've also seen patients who never recovered from major surgery for ovarian cancer. Sometimes it's not the cancer that ends their lives, it's the huge operation. Ask your doctor to explain the details of all treatments and what recovery will be like. Use the Best Case/Worst Case approach in making your decision.

Chemotherapy: Traditional chemotherapy tries to kill rapidly dividing cells. Since cancer cells tend to divide rapidly, they're susceptible to being killed by chemotherapy. Unfortunately, many normal, healthy cells also divide rapidly, including those that line your mouth, intestines, and hair follicles, and those in your bone marrow that make blood cells. Chemo can inflame the lining of your mouth and bowels and cause severe mouth pain and diarrhea. The killing of hair follicles can make your hair fall out. The impact on your bone marrow can lead to anemia, which can make you feel weak and put you at risk of bleeding and getting infections. All these side effects can be managed, but they take a toll. In addition, many chemotherapy agents cause severe nausea and vomiting. Fortunately, there are good medications that prevent and treat nausea. New cancer treatments are being developed all the time, and many have fewer side effects, but no treatment is risk-free.

Losing your hair or having some nausea is tolerable if the treatment shrinks your cancer and helps you achieve your goals. Despite the benefits of chemotherapy, you'll probably experience its toxic effects. If, even after chemo, your cancer has spread widely, the odds that more chemotherapy will provide any benefit are vanishingly small.

Radiation therapy: Radiation therapy works on the same principle as traditional chemotherapy. The radiation damages and kills rapidly dividing cells. The goal is to concentrate the radiation on the cancer, while causing as little damage as possible to the surrounding normal tissues. Of course, it's impossible not to hit some nearby tissues as the radiation goes through your body. To limit the damage to normal tissue, radiation for initial cancer treatment is divided into multiple parts or fractions and typically given daily for a number of weeks. The idea is to kill the cancer with radiation while giving the normal tissues around it time to recover. Your daily treatment may take only a few minutes, and you may not feel much of anything. In the early going, patients usually tell me, "Hey, this is easy." But before long, the side effects build up and take a toll.

Radiation focused on even a minuscule part of your body can make you feel bad all over. At the site of the radiation, skin can become inflamed and painful, as can the lining of your mouth. You can also become fatigued and lose your appetite. If the radiation hits your intestine, it can cause abdominal pain and diarrhea. Many side effects can be treated, some can be prevented, and all will pass with time.

When my grandmother had radiation for breast cancer, she initially said that the radiation was nothing, that it was easy compared to chemotherapy and surgery. But as the weeks went on, the skin over the area of the radiation got red, irritated, and painful, and my grandmother was exhausted. She could barely get out of bed to go for treatments. She couldn't understand what was happening. So I explained that the radiation was causing her painful skin, which made sense to her. I also told her that the radiation was causing her to be so tired, which made no sense to her at all. She couldn't believe that a treatment taking just a few minutes a day, that directed something invisible at her chest she couldn't even detect, could make her feel so awful.

Many weeks later, my grandmother regained her energy and her skin no longer hurt. Over time, she could barely remember the effects of the radiation. The treatments worked to cure her breast cancer, and what she had gone through was all a vague memory.

Radiation for bone pain from cancer: Sometimes radiation is used in advanced cancer, not to treat the original site of the cancer but to treat metastases, places where the cancer has spread and is causing symptoms. Some cancers, like lung cancer and breast cancer, have a tendency to spread to the bones. Cancer in the bones can be extremely painful and lead to fractures. Radiation can effectively reduce the pain. It is important to know that in this setting, a single dose or fraction of radiation is as effective as multiple fractions. The evidence is so strong that professional medical societies recommend single fraction radiation in these situations. A single fraction is easier, takes less time, and is as effective. If you're offered radiation for pain caused by cancer that has spread to your bones (bone metastases), you should demand single fraction radiation.

Ventricular assist devices: As I mentioned earlier, ventricular assist devices (VADs) are pumps surgically implanted in the chest and connected to the heart that help circulate your blood. They're used for patients whose hearts cannot pump enough blood for them to stay alive. VADs are most commonly used to help the left part of the heart, the part that pumps blood to your whole body, which is why I use the term LVAD, L for *left*. LVADs have a cable that is connected to a power source outside your body and are amazingly small and powerful. Some people may be too sick for an LVAD, and the operation to implant it could be too much for them. When an LVAD is surgically placed, it's permanent and can't be removed, but it can be disconnected. If it's disconnected, the patient's weak heart has to pump on its own, and death usually follows within about 15 minutes.

The operation to implant an LVAD is serious, and living with an LVAD isn't easy. Patients constantly worry that it might disconnect or malfunction. Recipients must take blood thinners to prevent clotting, and those thinners can lead to bleeding—including bleeding in the brain, which can be devastating. Patients with an LVAD who suffer catastrophic illness, such as a major stroke or an advanced cancer, often decide that their quality of life is so poor that they ask for their LVADs to be turned off.

Vincent, a sixty-two-year-old man, had advanced heart failure. His heart was so weak he could no longer walk more than a few steps before he became tired and short of breath. Despite trying numerous heart medications, he had to sleep sitting up or risk severe shortness of breath. His quality of life was miserable. He was admitted to the hospital, and it became clear that an LVAD would be a good option for him.

I met with Vincent to evaluate him for an LVAD. He told me an interesting story. It seems he had met with the social worker for the LVAD team, who explained what his life would be like with an LVAD and the risks associated with it. She said he would need someone with him all the time in case the battery pack became disconnected and that if he didn't take blood thinners religiously, his pump could clot off and he could die. She also warned that the blood thinners could cause bleeding in his brain that could be fatal.

After that conversation, Vincent wanted nothing to do with an LVAD. However, later that day, the surgeon who was to implant the LVAD stopped by and assured him that the LVAD was a great treatment. He also said that the surgery would be a piece of cake and that he was very confident that Vincent would survive surgery and the pump would perform well. The surgeon told Vincent not to worry.

Vincent decided to proceed. He was angry that the social worker had been so negative and caused him so much worry. He was also grateful to the surgeon for being so supportive and positive and for making the LVAD sound great.

Of course, the social worker and the surgeon were both right. For some patients, an LVAD will be wonderful, and at the same time, the risks and future lifestyle modifications are real. If you get conflicting information, try to bring all the parties together and speak with them at the same time. Have them explain the treatments in simple terms and point out the pros and cons. Ask questions, tell them your goals, and find out what you can reasonably expect.

Dialysis: Dialysis, which is one of the wonders of modern medicine, replaces the function of sick kidneys and removes toxins from the blood, balances salts, and removes excess water from the body. Two basic types of dialysis exist: hemodialysis, the most common type, and peritoneal dialysis. Hemodialysis does the work of the kidneys by circulating blood through a machine with a special filter. Hemodialysis patients typically go to a facility three times a week for two to three hours, during which their blood is continuously circulated through the machine. After hemodialysis treatments, patients may feel weak, tired, or dizzy. Hemodialysis is often used in hospitals when patients with serious illness develop kidney problems.

Prior to dialysis treatment, which became available in the 1960s, kidney failure meant certain death within weeks. At first, dialysis machines were so rare that committees were appointed to decide which kidney failure patients would get dialysis. Since dialysis was literally a matter of life or death, the first committee was dubbed the "God Committee." Today, access to dialysis in the developed world is unlimited, and in the United States, dialysis is the only medical intervention for which Medicare guarantees payment.

Peritoneal dialysis involves placing a catheter in the abdominal wall to allow large amounts of a special solution to be placed into the abdominal cavity. An advantage of peritoneal dialysis is that you can do it at home and don't have to go to a facility. It is also possible, though uncommon, to receive hemodialysis at home. The solution stays in for four to twelve hours and is then drained through the catheter. The solution contains concentrations of salts and other chemicals that help remove toxins from the blood. Patients who go through peritoneal dialysis typically infuse the solution several times a day, every day, or use a machine overnight while they sleep to circulate the fluid in and out of the abdomen. Peritoneal dialysis is never used in patients whose kidneys suddenly fail, which is common in hospitals, but is offered to those who gradually develop kidney failure.

Organ transplants: Transplants can be miraculous. For patients with liver, heart, or lung failure, they may offer the only chance for long-term survival. I've seen many patients who were at death's door gain a new lease on life after an organ transplant. Unfortunately, the demand for organs for transplants greatly outnumbers those available, and many people die waiting for them. Transplants are not without risk, and life with a transplant is not easy. Patients must diligently take numerous medications each day to prevent their bodies from attacking and rejecting their new organs. Medications to reduce rejection weaken the immune system and increase the risk of infections. Some new organs simply don't work well or work at all. Evaluating whether to have an organ transplant is a lengthy, rigorous, and involved process because transplants have significant risks, and the supply of organs to transplant is so limited.

Mechanical ventilation: When you're too sick to breathe on your own, a plastic tube can be placed down your throat and into your lungs, and connected to a machine that will breathe for you. Mechanical ventilation is most often used while you wait for your lungs to get well enough for you to resume breathing on your own. Unfortunately, failing lungs can be a sign that the body is shutting down, and when it is, mechanical ventilation, like hemodialysis for kidney failure in that setting, simply prolongs the inevitable. When you're receiving mechanical ventilation, you can't speak because the tube passes through your voice box. Often, you need to be sedated because the treatment is so uncomfortable. Mechanical ventilation can be lifesaving. If you suddenly develop lung failure and you're too sick to tell doctors and hospitals that you don't want mechanical ventilation or haven't specified it in writing, they'll assume that you want it. I discuss documenting your wishes in writing in greater detail in chapter 11.

For patients with conditions that cause muscle weakness, such as ALS, a ventilator may be needed when they get too weak to breathe. Usually, these patients have no expectation of improvement, but they would die without mechanical ventilation. Many ALS patients choose to have mechanical ventilation at home. Mechanical ventilation can be stopped when patients feel that it is no longer effective or their quality of life has become too poor.

RX

When my mom was diagnosed with lung cancer, we found out that she had a rare type that didn't typically respond to the usual chemotherapy. She was getting care at a local hospital in Los Angeles, where she lived, but I wanted her to come to UCSF for a second opinion with our lung cancer experts. I found studies that suggested that treatment for kidney cancer might work for my mom's cancer based on a similar genetic mutation and hoped my colleague could find something that would work.

My mom elected to get chemotherapy at her local hospital. After one treatment that caused her nausea and pain, she decided to stop. She knew that chemo couldn't cure her illness. She knew it made her sick. As much as I wanted her to come to UCSF, she felt too sick. Her goal was to be in her home with the big TV and new white carpet and to spend time with her family and friends. An exhausting trip to San Francisco and more chemo would only take away from that. Even with everything I knew about her illness, I found myself hoping we could find a treatment that would help. Not only did I need to accept the fact of my mom's illness and the reality of the situation, I also had to accept her choice. Looking back, she was so right. Somewhere she is smiling.

When it comes to treatments, people often use superlatives and classify them as either good or evil. They say that a certain treatment is evil, or great, or awesome, or horrible. "Don't do dialysis. It's just terrible." "Chemotherapy is evil. Avoid it if you can." "That operation was a godsend. You should have it." Those terms can influence your decisions. The same treatment may be a godsend for one person and the work of the devil for another. Giving treatments moral qualities can make them seem better or worse than they actually are.

Treatments, including surgery, chemotherapy, dialysis, LVAD, and others, are not imbued with moral character. They're tools that medical professionals use to help patients. Whether a treatment is right for you depends on you: your goals, your health, your condition, your hopes, your preferences.

chapter four

PROGNOSIS: WHAT DOCTORS SAY, WHAT THEY MEAN, AND WHAT PATIENTS HEAR

WHEN MOST PEOPLE GET A BAD DIAGNOSIS, THEIR FIRST thought is, "How long do I have?" It's often the first question they ask. Most are stunned; they're in a state of shock. Suddenly, their world has changed. What the brain briefly considered, and the heart could not accept, is now a fact: they're seriously ill. At this point, their minds go numb; they feel lost, completely in the dark. Their thoughts turn to the possibility of dying, and they instinctively ask how long they have.

People want to know their prognosis. They think, "OK, I've got cancer, heart failure, or dementia, what does that mean? What am I in for, what's in store?" And not surprisingly, we all want our prognosis to be good. People rush to the Internet for answers. Their minds run wild. They recall stories they've heard and what others went through. "Uncle Joe was diagnosed with cancer and died three weeks later." "Sam, my neighbor, went to the hospital for shortness of breath. The doctors said he had heart failure, and five days later he was dead." "My coworker was diagnosed with cancer twenty-five years ago. The doctors told him he had only a few months to live, but he's fit as a fiddle and the doctor has since died."

Each prognosis is specific to each person. What happened to others with your condition may or may not happen to you. Your situation could be better or worse.

> I had to tell Sam, a dear eighty-nine-year-old patient, that he had colon cancer. Sam immediately thought that he had only two or three weeks to live because his cousin, who had had the same illness, went fast. I told Sam that I thought he had more like a year. I shudder to think what might have happened had Sam left my office thinking he had only a few weeks left. He probably would have made premature decisions, some of which might have been rash. When I gave Sam my prognosis, he was relieved. Who would have thought that a prognosis of a year would be good news, but given his initial fear, it was a gift.

Although patients have the right to know their prognosis, doctors don't like to answer directly. Giving patients a poor prognosis is stressful, unpleasant, and gut wrenching, especially when patients and doctors have known each other long and well. Conversations about prognosis can make everyone feel bad.

I tell my students that the goal of prognosis conversations with patients is not to feel good, but to help patients understand reality and feel supported. Doctors should be kind and gentle, but also clear and direct.

Some people think that if they don't talk about difficult or sad matters, then they won't feel sad, but I disagree. It doesn't work that way. Bottling up our fears is stressful and saps our energy. If you think that talking about difficult matters won't help, you're wrong—it does.

Not discussing your prognosis doesn't mean that you're not thinking about it. Discussions can ease your concerns. They can also reveal useful information, and you may learn that your situation is better than you feared. When the news is worse, you can plan how to make the most of your situation.

When it comes to health, I'm a firm believer in talking about the hard stuff. I can't say that it won't be difficult or sad, but by then, it's usually already sad. When you're in the dark, without crucial information, you can stumble and make decisions you'll later regret. However, talking about your prognosis and getting the facts can relieve your stress, provide support, and help you make a strong plan for moving forward.

DOCTORS DISLIKE GIVING PROGNOSES

Doctors know that their seriously ill patients are fragile, and they don't want to cause them any more pain. If they give honest prognoses, they worry it will destroy their patients' hopes.

Sandy's breast cancer had spread to her bones, liver, lungs, and chest. Fluid around both lungs had to be drained by tubes to prevent her from being short of breath. She was weak, was bed bound, and barely ate. One morning after we got her symptoms controlled, I asked Sandy what her doctors had told her to expect. She told me that a month ago her doctor said that she had about *five years* to live. Her biggest concern was where she would live during those five years. I was shocked. Given her condition, I thought Sandy had about *two to three months* to live, and I was concerned about her false, unrealistic hopes.

Hope based on misinformation is not real hope, and ultimately, false hope is no hope. I gently told Sandy that while the five-year prognosis might have been true at some point, her condition had deteriorated, and I asked her if she wanted to know what I thought. She said, "Yes." Was she sad? Absolutely. Was she surprised? Not really. In fact, she admitted that she couldn't see how she could live another five years given how much weaker she had become.

Even with such a limited prognosis, Sandy had hope, realistic hope. Her housing problem was solved when she was invited to stay with a friend for the next few months through the end of her life. Sandy was eager to leave the hospital. Since her symptoms were well controlled, Sandy left the hospital and received hospice care at her friend's home.

Realistic prognoses focus hope. They give patients reliable and realistic information they can use to make decisions. Hope is important. It's such a significant factor in dealing with serious illness that I discuss it in detail in chapter 7. As it relates to prognosis, hope is not a reason to withhold prognostic information; it is a compelling reason to share it.

> Information about prognosis influences your decisions. It enables you to plan. When you know your prognosis, you can make life choices that may be more important than deciding whether to try a certain treatment. Information helps you think about and determine how and where you want to spend the time you have and with whom.

ASSUMPTIONS AND MISINTERPRETATIONS

Patients make assumptions based on what doctors say and don't say. If a doctor says, "Come back and see me in three months," most patients will logically assume that the doctor thinks that they will live at least another three months. Generally, that's a safe assumption. However, when patients are very sick, a doctor may tell them to schedule another visit simply out of habit or because she can't bear to tell them that she thinks they have less than that time left. It may just be easier for her to tell them to schedule another appointment.

While at home, Chen, an eighty-six-year-old man with heart failure, became very short of breath. He was hospitalized and fortunately did well. After a few days, he was well enough to go home. When I saw him in my office a week later, I explained that this episode could happen again if he wasn't careful about his medications and diet. Chen was quite concerned and committed to following doctors' orders.

I saw Chen three months later. His heart failure was under control, he was in good shape, and he was walking two miles a day. As we were talking, Chen said that he was planning to take his entire family—his wife, their three children and their spouses, and fourteen grandchildren—on a cruise to Alaska in June. I said that it sounded lovely. Then it occurred to me that it was January. Chen was not just telling me about his travel plans. He was asking if I thought he'd make it to June and be well enough to travel.

If I said nothing, he would tell his wife that he had mentioned the trip and I said, "Sounds lovely," which meant that I thought he'd be fine. If I was worried about him and didn't think he'd make it to June, I would have said something. I then asked Chen if he was worried that he might be too sick to travel or that he might not make it to June. He said, "Yes." He told me that he couldn't just ask, but he figured if I didn't say no, it meant he'd be fine.

The next time I saw Chen, we leafed through a stack of photos. In each, Chen and members of his family were beaming, savoring the cruise and their time together.

What sounded like innocuous travel plans was really an important prognosis question. As patients often do, Chen was asking me to give him a prognosis indirectly. Had I not figured out what Chen was actually asking, he probably would have guessed correctly from my reply.

Guessing, however, is dangerous because patients frequently guess wrong. They interpret, infer, and jump to conclusions. They often conclude that they have more or less time than they actually do.

Misunderstandings frequently occur when doctors outline treatment regimens with their patients. When doctors tell patients, "We'll give you a three-month cycle of chemo, take a month off, and then do another three-month cycle," patients instantly calculate that they have at least another seven months to live. At the same time, the doctor may be worried that the patient won't make it through the first chemo cycle.

 Don't guess. Knowing your prognosis is too important. And don't try to infer what your prognosis is from what your doctor says or doesn't say. Ask your doctor directly, "What's my prognosis?"

Patients assume that their doctors would never give them chemotherapy unless they thought it would shrink their cancer, that they would not operate unless they thought there was a good chance it would help, and that if they really thought someone was too sick for an LVAD, they would come right out and say so. Not true! Many doctors don't like to give poor prognoses. So doctors say, "If you get stronger, come to the clinic and we can give you chemo," knowing full well that the patient will only get sicker, not stronger. We tell patients that they're on the list for a liver transplant, knowing that they'll die before getting to the top of the list.

INFORMATION AND DECISIONS

The most important reason to know your prognosis is that you'll live your life differently when you learn how much remaining time you have. If you're told that you only have months to a year to live, you'll make different decisions than you otherwise would have. Conversely, when you believe that you have years to live, you will probably put off some important decisions because you think that you can make them later.

How and why we make decisions and use our time tends to be very functional and adaptable. At different times and during different circumstances, our focus, priorities, and needs change. For example, early in one's career, deeply focused work and very long hours may be necessary.

As a doctor, some of my training was brutal. During my internship, my first year after medical school, and my first year as a doctor, I worked long, extended hours. For several months, I spent every day caring for patients and every third night in the hospital. Out of the 168 hours in a week, I routinely worked more than 100.

Was it stressful? Yes.

Did I learn a lot? Yes.

Would I do it all over to become a doctor? Yes.

Would I spend the last year of my life that way? No way!

If you only have another year to live, you can plan to live it differently. Here's some of what I would do. I would:

> Spend more time with family and friends.
> Take that trip.
> Dig into the bucket list.
> Play more.
> Work less.
> Eat more ice cream.
> Write another book.

Some changes are profound, some are not. Some may not be for everyone but may have special significance for you. The point is that when you think your life will change and that your time is limited, you can adapt, plan, and adjust. You can make important, reality-based decisions. When you understand your prognosis, you'll know when it's time to act and what you most want to do.

Interestingly, I've found that many people who suddenly have a limited prognosis want nothing more than to return to the life they had before they were sick. They want to get back to work and to their familiar routines. They don't want their illnesses to alter their lives. And yet, even these people have a different attitude and approach. How could they not? When you're seriously ill, priorities shift, often in good ways. And if your prognosis turns out to be much longer than you initially expected, how wonderful! You've made the changes that most of us would love to make but can't seem to manage, and you have longer to enjoy them.

I don't mean to say that a limited prognosis is a good thing. Living longer is better. But that's not the issue. The real issue is that if you're in a situation in which your prognosis is limited, it's helpful to know that and to have as much good information about it as possible.

We all differ. Some people don't want to know their prognosis. Or they don't want to talk about it. That's perfectly fine. It's their lives and their decisions. Some find comfort in uncertainty or feel that their prognosis is too difficult to discuss. Others just prefer not knowing. I respect their feelings and their right to make those decisions.

DISCUSSING PROGNOSIS

Yogi Berra is credited with saying, "Prediction is hard, especially of the future." As with many sayings attributed to Yogi, this one rings true. Making predictions is hard. Numerous factors are involved that can vary from person to person and case to case.

> When patients ask about prognosis, doctors may not know the answers. They certainly don't know precisely what will happen, when it will occur, and all that will be involved.
> Prognoses are based on statistics, averages of how long people with the same illnesses lived, and our experience. Older doctors are better at prognostication. But since those statistics are based on averages and patient populations, they don't take into account a patient's specific characteristics or provide very precise information.

› Some doctors are concerned about self-fulfilling prophecies. They're afraid that talking about a limited prognosis could make it come true.

Here is what is true about prognoses:

1. Prognostication is inherently uncertain. We can't predict exactly what will happen to any one person and when it will occur.
2. Doctors usually have more information than they share.
3. Information does not have to be precise to be valuable. Knowing that winter is the rainy season and that summer is dry is helpful in planning a vacation, even though we don't know the exact forecast for the days we plan to travel six months from now.

Doctors know that some people beat the averages, while others fall short. They've also seen the extremes: cases where the most unlikely candidates defy all expectations to survive, and the rapid demise of those who seemed less seriously ill. And they usually can't explain the reasons for these outcomes. Some differences may be attributable to the biology of the illness and the biology of the individual because they interact in subtle and important ways that we don't fully understand.

A lot is involved in prognosis discussions. Some doctors excel in explaining information clearly and in answering your questions to make sure you understand. Others are notorious for not doing it well. Some patients don't want all the details. They trust their doctors and will unquestioningly accept their recommendation. If you want enough information to make the best possible decision, press your doctors for clarification. Find out what they actually know and think and make sure that you truly understand what they say.

ASKING ABOUT YOUR PROGNOSIS

You have the right to know your prognosis. So simply ask your doctor directly, "How long do you think I have?" If your doctor says, as so many do, "Who can really know?" or "I don't have a crystal ball," it's a cop-out. While both those statements are true, they're also meaningless. These evasive answers don't help patients. They may, in fact, be a disservice that keeps seriously ill people from making the most of their time.

If your doctor hesitates or is reluctant to be specific, explain that you understand that he or she can't give you a precise date and time but that you'd appreciate a range, such as days to weeks, weeks to months, months to years, or a few years. Showing your understanding can ease your doctor's reluctance and discomfort.

Your doctor should be able to give you a range. If your doctor still demurs, ask for best- and worst-case ranges. Ask about statistics, studies, and his or her experience.

When I teach doctors to give patients' prognoses, I suggest that they put them in ranges. Providing ranges acknowledges that the prognosis is inherently uncertain but that the doctor is trying to be helpful by giving his or her best guess.

Beware of anyone who gives you a specific amount of time, such as, "I think you probably have six months." Doctors can't predict with such accuracy and are certain to be wrong. Ask your doctor to clarify: "Do you mean six months to a year?"

My UCSF colleagues Drs. Eric Widera and Alex Smith and others developed the website ePrognosis (eprognosis.ucsf.edu) to provide prognostic information for doctors and patients. They scoured the medical literature to provide the best studies and information available. ePrognosis includes several indexes for calculating prognosis. Some accurately predict survival over the next several years, while others have shorter time horizons. However, the ranges are usually broad.

> If your doctor isn't forthcoming about your prognosis, press him or her for information about it—even when it may be hard to get. You have a right to know what your doctor knows. Understanding your prognosis and what the future may look like is important. It will influence the decisions you make.

WHAT DOCTORS SAY AND WHAT THEY MEAN

Knowing your prognosis is crucial. It's a critical piece of information that you need to plan your treatment—and, more important, to plan your life. Discussing your prognosis and treatment can be difficult for both patients and doctors. At the same time, these are crucial conversations because the stakes are high and the truth can help.

Communication problems exist in medicine, not because doctors want to withhold or be evasive, but because we have to talk about matters that are sad and complex with people who are grieving and facing loss. It's not the most ideal scenario.

Talking about prognosis and other complex topics with patients isn't easy for doctors. They have to choose their words carefully and proceed cautiously with what they say and how they say it. Until recently, most doctors weren't taught how to talk to patients about prognosis and other thorny subjects in medical school or during their residencies. They learned on the job, and in the process they made mistakes and picked up bad habits.

Conversations about prognosis are awkward and uncomfortable for patients and their families. They don't discuss prognosis freely around the dinner table. Frequently, patients and their families don't understand what doctors and nurses tell them or the language they use. Since that language can be highly technical and opaque, it should come as no surprise that when doctors and patients talk, important information gets lost and misunderstood.

In the pages that follow, I identify common communication problems that cause information to be unclear, confusing, and misunderstood. I also discuss what doctors say and what they mean, and what patients and their families hear and how they interpret what doctors say, and I suggest what you can do to avoid misunderstandings.

Jargon: When health professionals speak with patients, they can be bafflingly technical. They frequently talk in code and use language that patients can't understand. Often, this language is natural for them; it's what they use with colleagues and in their work. Doctors also speak in code when they're uncomfortable and are afraid that the patient can't handle the truth.

As in all businesses and professions, medicine has its own unique technical language, or jargon. It's an insiders' language that's also called medicalese and doctor-speak. Jargon is shorthand we learn in medical and nursing school and use with our colleagues to communicate precisely and efficiently. A single word or short phrase can quickly convey complex information, processes, and procedures.

Medical students embrace jargon and make it part of their vocabularies. Using jargon gives them status; it identifies them as medical practitioners, members of an admired and respected profession.

A good example of jargon is the word *ambulate*. Most people never use the word, but doctors and nurses do so routinely. They inquire whether a patient can ambulate. *Ambulate* is health professionals' jargon for "get around" and includes walking but is more than that. Trouble is, if a doctor or nurse tells a family member that their mother needs to ambulate three times a day, you'd have to wonder what the family would think.

Health care professionals constantly use jargon. It becomes second nature to us. We use it so frequently in our work that it slips into our conversations with our patients and their families and with our families and friends. We even use it when we're not talking about medicine.

I once heard a colleague say that she was getting a "bolus" of visitors for the holidays. Now, bolus is defined as follows:

a. A rounded mass; a large pill; a soft mass of chewed food; a dose of a substance (as a drug) given intravenously
b. A large dose of a substance given by injection for the purpose of rapidly achieving the needed therapeutic concentration in the bloodstream

Notice that neither definition relates to a group of people. In medicine, *bolus* is usually definition *b*: a large amount of a substance, typically salt water or medicine, given at once or rapidly. When my colleague referred to a bolus of visitors, she meant a group of people coming over at the same time. Only health care workers would use that word to mean lots of visitors at once.

As a palliative care physician, I work with patients who have many different illnesses. Those patients are treated by other doctors who specialize in a wide array of fields. Frequently, I'm not familiar with the jargon those specialists use, and I find myself asking them to explain what they said in plain English.

Do the same. When someone, anyone—doctors, nurses, or anyone else—uses jargon that you don't understand, put up your hand, stop them, and ask them to explain what they mean in language that you can easily understand. Asking for explanations doesn't mean you're stupid. In fact, it shows that you're smart and engaged. *Mechanical ventilation*, *intubation*, *sepsis*, *pressors*, *diuresis*, and *febrile* are all jargon—medical language that nonclinicians should not be expected to understand.

I teach my students never to use jargon with patients and their families. Instead, I suggest that they speak plainly and directly and use language that patients and their families will understand. I also suggest that they ask patients and their families if everything they said is clear and ask what questions they have.

I understand that avoiding jargon is tough. It often requires breaking deeply entrenched, often long-standing habits. Explaining technical matters isn't easy, and it's particularly difficult to do to those who are worried and upset. However, when doctors speak with patients and their families, they must be clear and make sure that they are fully understood.

Here are some other common phrases that can be easy to misinterpret but are important for you to understand:

Positive: The word *positive* usually means "good." We like positive attitudes, positive states of mind, and positive balance sheets. However, in medicine, positive is often bad. A positive lymph node means cancer is in a lymph node and has spread. Positive biopsy margins signify that not all the cancer was removed and some remains in the body. Positive blood cultures mean bacteria are growing in a patient's blood, which is potentially life threatening within hours if not promptly treated. When a skin test for tuberculosis is positive, it means you've been exposed to tuberculosis and could harbor that dreaded disease. A positive CT scan could mean that you have a blood clot in your lung. Though we think of negative things as being bad, in these examples, negative would be great.

I first encountered this confusion during medical school, at the height of the AIDS epidemic in relation to HIV. I remember a patient asking me why the term "HIV positive" means you're infected with what was then a fatal virus. Having HIV felt negative; calling it positive seemed like a cruel joke.

To avoid potential confusion, I tell my students not to use the word *positive*. Instead, I suggest that they state what it is:

> There is bacteria in the blood that indicates a very serious infection.
> We found cancer in the lymph node, which means that the cancer has spread beyond the lung.
> The biopsy showed that we didn't get all the cancer; some is left behind and will require another operation.
> The CT scan showed that you have a blood clot in the lung that needs immediate treatment.

If your doctor says that something is positive, *get clarification. Ask, "Is it good positive or bad positive?" and then have your doctor explain.*

Progress: Much like the word *positive*, *progress* usually denotes something good. Normally, it means moving forward, getting better, advancing in a productive way. In medicine, progress and progression can be bad. When cancer progresses it means it is spreading, and more cancer is always worse. When heart disease progresses, it means the heart is weaker. A progressive disease marches on and keeps getting worse. On the other hand, making progress in the ICU means that you are getting better.

If you hear your doctor use the word progress *or* progressive, *ask her what she means. Are things getting better or worse?*

Response: "Response" and "response rates" are terms used in describing the effectiveness of chemotherapy. Oncologists repeatedly use them when they discuss specific treatments. However, the word *response* doesn't necessarily mean what you think.

What does it mean when a doctor says, "This treatment has a 30 percent response rate"? You might reasonably think that it means that the treatment cured 30 percent of those who received it. What it really means is that in 30 percent of the people who took the treatment, the cancer showed no growth or actually got smaller.

To further complicate matters, there are different types of responses: a "complete response" and a "partial response." A complete response, which indicates that all detectable cancer is gone, may signify a cure, but not necessarily. It means that the chemo worked to reduce the cancer so it's undetectable on a scan. However, undetectable microscopic areas of cancer may still exist and could grow back.

A partial response means that the cancer has shrunk by at least 50 percent. A partial response is good news, but not as good as a complete response. Of course, a 30 percent response rate is the same as a 70 percent no-response rate, but we never word it that way, even though studies show that people choose differently depending on how statistical information is presented.

If your doctor talks to you about response rates, ask her to explain it in plain language. What does she mean by response? *What kind of response?*

Survival: The issue here is not with the word *survival*. In medicine, like in any other setting, survival means being alive. And that's a good thing. The challenge is that doctors have different ways of talking about survival as it relates to a group of people who received a certain treatment. The "overall survival" rate is the percentage of cancer patients who are alive at some period of time after they began treatment. Typically, overall survival is measured in years: one, two, five, or ten. Although the overall survival rate may be the best measure of a treatment's success and the one you care about most, many treatment studies don't last long enough to report overall survival.

Another common and confusing term is "median survival." In calculating how long people live after they receive a certain treatment for a serious condition where death is common, researchers often report the "median survival," which is the length of time after treatment when only half of the group is still alive. A median survival of ten months means that only half the patients were still alive ten months after they entered the study.

It's important to know the overall survival and median survival rates for patients who received treatment and compare them with the rates for patients who didn't get treatment. If the difference is only a month or two, you may not want to spend them receiving chemotherapy and feeling sick.

Ask your doctor about median survival and overall survival for people with your condition. Also ask about median and overall survival with and without the treatment you're considering. You may find that survival for those who received the treatment was longer— but not long enough to be worthwhile.

"Would you like us to do everything possible?" I hear this question all the time in the hospital. Doctors frequently ask it to patients and their families. The problem is that it's a bad question because the only possible answer is "Yes." I've never heard any-one say "No."

When doctors say "everything possible," they are referring to a dizzying and frightening arsenal of interventions and invasive procedures. In my experience, when patients consent, they don't envision all the possibilities, some of which could be extensive and potentially harmful.

I teach my students never to ask this question. Any question that has only one answer—which may not be the right answer—is a bad question. Instead, I suggest that they ask, "How were you hoping we could help?"

Mrs. Chan was eighty-nine years old and had widely spread, metastatic ovarian cancer. She was living at home with her son and daughter-in-law and enrolled in home hospice. One morning the family came in to check on her and found her laboring to breathe and moaning. They panicked. Instead of calling hospice, they called 911. Mrs. Chan was rushed to the hospital. The ER doctor, confronted by a dying patient whom he didn't know, had to act quickly. He asked the family, "Would you like us to do everything possible?" to which they of course said, "Yes."

The ER launched into battle mode. Mrs. Chan was prepared for the ICU, and the big artillery was rolled out: large-caliber IVs, blood-drawing equipment, oxygen, X-rays, and a ventilator. Medical teams were called to enter the battle. My colleague and mentor was on call for the medical team. He heard about Mrs. Chan and ran down to the ER to see her and meet her family. He immediately put a hold on the interventions and quickly gathered the family.

"Your mom is very sick," he said.

"Yes, we know."

"How were you hoping we could help?"

"She is dying and we want you to help her." Her son held up a paper bag and said, "We want to dress her in these new clothes for her journey to the next world."

"We can use medicine to help her feel better and calmer. You can dress her in her new clothes right here in the ER. We will then move her to a quiet room upstairs where all of you can be with her for her final hours."

"Thank you."

Mrs. Chan died a few hours later—peacefully, surrounded by twenty family members, and looking lovely in her new clothes.

If a doctor asks if you want everything done, feel free to answer, "Of course I want everything done that will help me achieve my goals. Let me tell you what my goals are." Explain what you hope to achieve and what is important to you. Then talk with the doctor about which treatments will help you reach your goal.

Dignity: When patients are nearing death, doctors often use "dignity" as a code word and reason to stop all treatments, disconnect the machines, and let patients die. They often tell patients' loved ones, "We should focus on your mom's dignity," without going into specific details. Usually, what they mean is that the patient should no longer be subjected to the indignity of being unable to function and of being kept alive by artificial means.

When doctors speak of dignity, they often convey the impression that a universal dignity standard exists, which it does not. The meaning of dignity is subjective; it differs from patient to patient, loved one to loved one, and doctor to doctor. As a result of their illnesses, seriously ill patients may define dignity differently than they did before. And due to their hopes and love for the patient, families' definitions also may evolve.

If you're seriously ill, tell your family and friends what dignity means to you. If your loved one has a serious illness, ask what dignity means to him or her. If doctors and nurses say they want to respect your dignity, ask them precisely what they mean.

Withdrawal of care: If you or your loved one is in the ICU, being kept alive by machines, and despite all measures the situation turns dire, a decision may be made to "withdraw care." This means stopping the medicines and machines that have been keeping the patient alive, and letting him or her die peacefully and naturally. My problem with this language is that we should never withdraw care. We may withdraw certain treatments, but we must always care for our patients.

When the decision is made to stop the machines and other treatments, I explain clearly what we're doing and emphasize that we will continue providing care. For example, we may tell a patient's loved ones, "We will stop the breathing machine and remove the tube from her throat. We will continue to give her medicine to make sure she is comfortable. We will remove the big IV line in her neck and the one in her wrist and take out the tube from her nose. We'll monitor her closely to make sure she is comfortable and treated with dignity."

When doctors tell you, "We're going to withdraw care," you'll know what they mean. They're going to stop the machines. But then say, "You'll still care for her," and ask, "What will you do to make sure she's comfortable?"

"There's nothing more we can do." I find this statement sad and untrue. It's sad because it leaves patients without any help at a vulnerable time, and it's untrue because it tells patients that they can't be helped, which is patently false. Something can always be done to make things better.

When doctors make this statement, they are trying to say that they can't cure the illness or slow it down. While that may well be true and it's important to be honest, saying "There's nothing more we can do" can leave patients feeling abandoned at the time they may need us the most.

Some doctors say that there's nothing more we can do when desperate patients beg for one more treatment, one more round of chemo, one more operation—anything to eke out a cure, slow down the illness, and prolong life. I've seen doctors and patients end up in a tug-of-war, with patients saying that there must be something more they can do and doctors insisting that there isn't.

I was asked to see a thirty-two-year-old man with cancer of the intestine. Numerous chemotherapy cycles had not slowed his cancer. His bowels were blocked; he was nauseated, vomiting, and on strong pain medications; and he could no longer get out of bed. I went to see him with the oncologist. The patient was so weak he could barely talk, so his father did most of the talking for him. He asked what else could be done to help his son.

The oncologist said, "There's nothing more we can do." At which point they began a tug of war. The father asked about more chemo. The oncologist said that there isn't any more, which the father would not accept.

"With so many chemo medicines, there must be something you could give my son."

"No. There isn't any more chemo to give," the doctor answered.

"What about radiation? They use radiation for cancer."

"I'm afraid not. It would hurt the bowel too much."

"But he's dying—why not just try it?"

"We just don't use it in this setting."

"What about cutting the cancer out?"

"No, that won't work either."

They went back and forth with no end in sight, and the conversation was getting more heated. So I interrupted, saying, "I *wish* there were some treatment that would make this cancer go away. But unfortunately there isn't. However, we have lots of things we can do to help. How about we focus on what we can do to help your son feel better?"

The father turned to me. His face softened, and his glare disappeared.

"Really? Like what?"

"Well, let's talk about what you both hope will happen at this point. I think there's a lot more we can do to make him comfortable, to help him be more alert so he can talk with his family and friends, and I think, if he and you want it, we can get him home to be closer to his loved ones."

His father relaxed. We all dropped the rope, and the tug of war ended. Now we were all on the same side.

The patient wanted to go home. So we replaced the tube in his nose with one that went directly into his stomach and was more comfortable. It also didn't frighten his children. We got his pain under control and gave him medicine to help him stay awake more. Then we arranged for him to go home and get good home care. As it turned out, there was a lot more we could do.

If a doctor ever tells you, "There's nothing more we can do," stop her and say, "Do you mean there's nothing more you can do to make my disease go away? If so, what can we do to help me feel better?"

The most important message to take away from this chapter—and from this book—is that something can always be done to help. Always.

RX

I teach my students to say, "I wish . . . " when patients ask for something that we can't provide, like a cure. What I like most about "I wish . . . " is that it's true. I truly wish we had treatments that would cure your cancer, strengthen your heart, or improve your lungs or memory. I would like nothing more than to make all diseases go away; it's a large part of why I became a doctor. But medicine and biology have limits. The reason we don't offer a cure for a particular disease is not because we don't want to give it but because medicine hasn't come up with it yet. Hopefully, we will one day soon. Unfortunately, that day will come too late for many. In the meantime, we can do a great deal to make bad situations better. We can focus on what we *can* do.

Don't be afraid to ask your doctor to clarify anything you don't understand. And don't be afraid to ask what else can be done to help you feel better. If your doctor doesn't have good ideas or the information you need, ask for a referral to one who might. The stakes are too high, and the truth is too important.

PART II

moving on and
getting through

chapter five

MANAGING YOUR MEDICAL CARE

To get the best medical care, be an active participant in your care. Health care is not like air travel, where the pilot flies the plane and you just sit back and relax. As a patient, you have to be more involved. You must be more like a copilot who has access to vital information that your doctor doesn't have.

You can monitor how you feel better than anyone else because you know yourself best. No one else knows exactly how you feel, when your symptoms started, your energy level, or how your medications are affecting you. Other people, including your doctors and medical team, may sympathize, they may have even had similar experiences, but they can't feel or quantify *your* experience. Nor can your family—even though they love you and they're paying close attention.

You know your body, how you're feeling, and when you're off your game. You can detect tiny changes, subtle nuances that others may never even notice. That knowledge and awareness can be critically important to your medical team.

When my father-in-law was undergoing treatment for colon cancer, he learned to monitor his condition and to be proactive in the management of his medical care. He was taking chemo-therapy that affected his blood count. When he felt tired and weak, he knew that his blood count had dipped too low and that it was time to get a blood transfusion. The transfusions always helped him feel better.

One time, while he was getting a transfusion, instead of feel-ing better, he felt worse. So he told the nurse. She said, "I'm running the blood in as fast as I can so we can get you out of here." My father-in-law knew that every other transfusion he received went slowly, so he told the nurse, "That may be the problem, please slow it down." At first, the nurse was reluctant, but my father-in-law, who was not shy about expressing what was on his mind, insisted. The nurse slowed down the infusion of blood, and my father-in-law felt much better.

How you feel is important; it's inside information that you alone possess. Use what you know, be proactive, and help your providers help you feel better. The information you give them can be crucial in diagnosing and treating your illness.

Although we now have the benefit of remarkable testing methods such as MRIs, PET scans, and CT scans, plus genetic testing, the most important information in diagnosing your condition comes from you: your history, your feelings, and your ability to function—to bathe, cook, dress, and care for yourself. When we speak with patients to compile data that we use in making diagnoses, we usually have the key information we need by the time the patient has finished telling us her history. Then we use tests to confirm or rule out our diagnoses.

When you meet with providers, don't hold back. It's not the time to be silent or shy. Instead, be forthcoming; tell the full story.

Fill them in on anything that could be related to your health, even if it seems insignificant or doesn't seem to make sense. You may have to tell the story a few times. Share what you think is going on and what you are worried about, but don't let the doctor fixate on your self-diagnosis. You may even need to ask the doctor specifically what else he thinks might be going on.

When I was a medical student on the cardiology service, I cared for Mr. Paxton, a seventy-one-year-old man with heart failure. He had swelling and pain in his feet, more in his left foot than his right. It was a familiar story. Mr. Paxton had been admitted many times with worsening heart failure and swollen feet. The ER doctor gave Mr. Paxton diuretics and admitted him. We continued the diuretics, but his swelling didn't get better, and his pain got worse.

Mr. Paxton told us he had never been in such pain. He said that his pain didn't feel like heart failure; he knew how that felt. I reported this to my resident, who said we had to go back to the patient and figure this out. So we talked with Mr. Paxton and examined him again. He had pain in the left ankle, with swelling and redness around the ankle but not the foot. And his right foot and ankle were fine.

Then my resident looked up and asked Mr. Paxton if he'd ever had gout. "Why yes, I have, but not for many years." Gout flare-ups resolve with or without treatment, though treatment makes them go away faster and can keep them from coming back. And gout is extremely painful, so shortening an episode and preventing others is important. As it turned out, Mr. Paxton's worsened heart failure was actually gout, and I learned a very important lesson about listening to patients.

Tell your physicians how you feel in detail. They're trained listeners who know the questions to ask and how to look for and pick up clues. They are adept at sifting information and identifying the bits and pieces that could help. And don't stop until you've told your story. Don't let the doctor settle on a diagnosis too quickly or cut you off too soon.

When providers take careful histories and ask key questions, critical information is usually disclosed. Sometimes the exact diagnosis may not be immediately apparent, but further down the line, the new information helps.

When I met with Bernardo, a thirty-eight-year-old insurance adjuster in urgent care, I was puzzled. He had no fever and didn't seem sick. He had come to urgent care on his own steam, he looked healthy, and his voice was clear and strong. He complained of having had a fever for a week that wouldn't go away. It all started with what seemed like a usual cold, with a runny nose, congestion, a mild cough, and a slight headache. Over a few days, most of Bernardo's symptoms seemed to get better, and his pulse and blood pressure were stable, but his fever and cough remained. I examined him and didn't find anything unusual except for some crackly sounds in his chest that I thought were probably just the remnants of his cold.

I told Bernardo that the cough and fever were most likely due to his cold, which was just taking its time going away, and that he'd be fine in a few more days. But he was insistent that something else was going on. "Doctor," he said, "didn't you hear me? I *had* a cold and got better, but this cough stuck around and is getting worse, and I'm having fevers, up to 102 degrees. I've had many colds. I don't think this is just a cold." As I listened to Bernardo, I realized he was right. It wasn't just a cold. When he told me his story again and I put it together with the sounds in his chest, I realized he might have pneumonia, an infection of the lung that can follow a cold.

Instead of sending Bernardo home, I sent him for a chest X-ray, which showed that he did in fact have pneumonia. I called him back into the exam room and said that he was exactly right; this was not just a cold. I thanked him for being insistent and gave him a prescription for antibiotics. He was a good advocate for himself—the way we all should be.

Since your history is so vital, help your medical team by giving them as much information as you can. The first time you meet a new doctor, tell the whole story from the time you last felt well to the present. Take them through the stages of your illness, including all the developments and aches and pains. Describe your symptoms and explain what makes you feel better and what makes you feel worse. Take all the time you need to fully detail what's going on. You should expect your doctor to review your medical record before your visit and to know the basics. But there is no substitute for you telling your story directly.

I teach my students to start their information-seeking conversations with patients by asking an open-ended question that doesn't simply have a yes or no answer. For example, they could ask, "How have things been going?" They should then listen to the answer and not speak for at least two minutes to let the patient provide more information. For busy doctors, two minutes can feel like an eternity, but it's not really very long. I ask my students to resist the temptation to interrupt.

> Doctors are responsible for asking their patients the right open-ended questions, listening carefully, and taking a complete history. Patients are responsible for providing full and accurate stories.

An analysis by Howard Beckman and Richard Frankel [5.1] of tape recordings of office visits found that, on average, physicians interrupted patients after only eighteen seconds. That's not a long time to talk or tell your story. Try it at home. Have someone interrupt you after only eighteen seconds. You'll see that it's definitely not enough time to say very much.

Before you speak with your medical team, make a written list of what you want to say. Start with your major concerns, the issues that are most important to you. In conversations, we tend to lead with the easy stuff, which may not be the most important information. We save the hard stuff for later, when we know that the person we're talking to is listening and really wants to hear what we have to say.

What if your doctor interrupts? Politely suggest that you would like to finish your story. Get back on track, stick to the facts, and don't wander. If your pain started three days ago while you were walking the dog uphill, that's important. However, it's not important for the doctor to know your dog's breed or why you decided to go to the park instead of around the block.

Most physicians are pressed for time; they try to keep on schedule. They want to see every patient and see him or her on time. So give them the most important information first. It's OK to start with a bit of casual conversation; the relationship between patients and doctors is personal and intimate and doesn't have to be all business. But be mindful of your doctor's time and use your time wisely to say what's on your mind and to get the information you need.

Your doctor may ask you to prioritize your list and suggest saving the less important or less urgent items for your next visit. So clearly explain what's bothering or concerning you most. Then the doctor will usually ask you questions based on your illness, treatment, and medications. While these questions are quite important, your agenda should come first.

A lot of the information about your condition and how you've been feeling should be collected at home. Write it all in a notebook or in a document on your computer, tablet, or phone. Check and update your records daily.

Keep track of how you're feeling and what you're going through. You don't need a minute-by-minute record of every day, but the details describing what you're experiencing can be very helpful. In your notes, describe:

> Your symptoms in detail. List whatever is bothering you. Try to be specific.
> How your symptoms have unfolded over time. Include when they started and when they worsened.
> What makes your symptoms better and what makes them worse.
> Anything else you notice, such as changes in weight, energy, eating, sleep, or how your clothes fit.
> The degree of your pain and discomfort on a scale of 0 to 10, with 10 being the worst (see chapter 6 for a detailed discussion about managing pain and other symptoms). Record the following about your pain:
   ◦ When you have it.
   ◦ How often you have it.
   ◦ How long it lasts.

- What you do about it (take medicines, use heat or ice, rest, meditate, etc.).
- Where it is and if it moves around.
- What it feels like. Is it sharp, dull, throbbing, or radiating? Is it cramping or squeezing? Do you feel burning or pins and needles? Is there numbness with the pain?
- How it limits you. What are you unable to do because of your pain? Can you drive, sit for more than twenty minutes, or bend? Has your activity level changed? Can you still walk to the corner store or up a flight of stairs? Do you have to stop along the way, when you used to be able to go the whole way?
- If a treatment worked, how long it lasted. What we call a placebo effect often occurs, and it's very powerful and real. Often, people will feel better and have less pain and less shortness of breath after the first dose or two of a medicine. Over the next few doses, the medication may no longer help because the effect was primarily based on the person's belief that it would work, not because of the medication's physiologic effect. That doesn't mean that it was "all in the patient's head," but it does mean that it probably won't be the right medicine long-term.

› Record keeping is important:
- Keep track of how you feel after taking a medicine. First, if you're having pain, record how severe it is on a 0 to 10 scale, with 10 being the worst. You might find it easier to rate it as none, mild, moderate, or severe. No monitors or tests can determine how much pain you are having; quantifying your pain can come only from you. Then note the time of day, what you're doing at the time (eating, resting, walking, bathing), and how much

of the medicine you've taken. About thirty minutes later, record the pain level again and how tired you feel. That's what we do in the hospital to monitor pain and figure out exactly how much medicine to give and how often. Bring this record to the doctor or email it to her. She can use it to tailor treatment to your needs.

- If you have heart failure, weigh yourself every day. Rapid changes in weight—a pound or two in a few days—are due to changes in the amount of fluid in your body. If your weight goes up, it means you're holding on to water, which can overwhelm your heart and suddenly worsen your heart condition. Too much fluid in your body can lead to shortness of breath that may require a visit to the ER and admission to the hospital. By monitoring your weight, you can keep track of your condition and plan what to do if your weight goes up. For example, you and your doctor can figure out your base weight when you don't have extra fluid. This is called your dry weight. You can then get directions for taking more diuretics (water pills) if your weight goes up to a certain level and go back to your usual dose once your weight comes down. If your weight doesn't go down or you get more short of breath despite taking more diuretics, alert your doctor.

Mr. Shabback had very advanced heart failure. He was admitted to the hospital with shortness of breath that was caused by excess fluid. We treated him with high doses of diuretics. He lost fifteen pounds of water in three days and felt better. He was at his dry weight. I told him to weigh himself every day, and if his weight went up by two pounds to double his diuretic dose.

A week later, I saw Mr. Shabback back in the hospital. He was short of breath again and had gained back ten pounds. I asked him what happened. Had he been weighing himself? He said, "Yes, every day." Did he notice his weight going up? "Yes." Did he take more diuretics? "No." Why not? He explained that his weight hadn't gone up by more than two pounds in a day, so he hadn't taken more medicine.

I realized that it was my fault for giving poor guidance, and I've used this lesson to emphasize the importance of giving clear and precise instructions.

Chart 5.1 illustrates the records you should maintain. List the date, time, pain level, activity, medicine, and response.

CHART 5.1

Date	Time	Pain level	Activity	Medicine/ response
3/10/16	10 am	8	Watching TV	Morphine 4 mg and heating pad
"	10:30 am	4	"	—
"	1 pm	7	Eating lunch	Morphine 4 mg
"	1:30 pm	3	Reading	Heating pad

Monitoring can be taken to an extreme. Follow your doctor's instructions, and don't overdo it. In general, checking your blood pressure and pulse daily is unnecessary. If you don't have heart failure, you don't need to check and record your weight daily—it won't change that quickly.

Another bodily function worth tracking, especially if you're taking opioids, is your bowel movements. More than three days without a bowel movement is a problem, and more than five days is a big problem. If you're taking opioids, take something to keep your bowels moving. Prunes and prune juice often work. There are many medications that can help keep things moving. Avoid fiber supplements, which are fine when you're not using opioids, but when you are, they can make your stool harder to pass.

If you're receiving chemotherapy or radiation, keep records of the dates and times you received your treatments and how and when you responded to those treatments.

> Did you get nauseated after chemo? If so, when and how bad was it?
> What medicines provided the most relief?
> What else did you do to relieve your nausea?
> Were you fatigued? If so, for how long?

This information can help you plan for future chemo cycles and help your doctor minimize possible side effects. If you're told to measure your fever at certain times, do it. Take your temperature and write it down along with the date and time. Then when you report that information to your doctors, better decisions can be made, decisions based on accurate information about your health.

MEDICATIONS

If you took a medication and experienced side effects, note when they started, how long they lasted, and their impact on you. Be as detailed and exacting as you can.

If you see consistent patterns, that's really important. Some "side effects" are not really that—they're just how you happened to feel that day, not a consistent reaction.

When you take a medication, every side effect does not necessarily indicate that you're allergic to those meds. I see many patients who report being allergic to a medicine, but when we talk, they report having unpleasant feelings after taking the medicine or that it didn't work as expected, which may not be a true allergy. If you get a rash, swelling of the lips, or itching, it generally means you shouldn't take that medicine or one from the same class.

Knowing what you're allergic to and making sure it's documented clearly in your medical record is crucial. You absolutely don't want to receive a medicine you are allergic to! However, true allergies to a medicine are much less common than situations in which patients don't respond to a medicine or don't like them. It's important to distinguish a true allergy from a milder reaction so that you don't unnecessarily exclude a medicine or class of medicines that might be important for you in the future.

Judy, a woman in her forties, had very serious lung disease. When we first met, she told me that she couldn't tolerate yellow pills. Any other colored pills were OK. She didn't react adversely to other colors, but yellow pills always made her ill. At first, I didn't believe it. How could that possibly be? How could she have a bad reaction to a color? I prescribed a small dosage of a new medicine. It was yellow. Judy called me to say she didn't want to take it. I convinced her to try since she really needed the medicine.

Sure enough, Judy had a real and consistent adverse reaction. I was baffled and never could explain this reaction, since yellow coloring is made in different ways. Nonetheless, we always had to make sure to avoid giving Judy yellow pills, and I would write on the prescription, "NO YELLOW PILLS."

The smartphone app epocrates (www.epocrates.com) describes medicines, dosages, side effects, and interactions with other medicines and also includes pictures. Whenever I pre-scribed a new medicine for Judy, we would look on my phone, check its color, and avoid those that were yellow. Judy could look at the picture on the app and tell me if it was yellow enough to cause a problem.

WHAT TO DO

Carry a list of all your medications on your person, on your smart-phone, in your wallet, or in your purse. Include the strength, how much and how often you take them. Make sure the list is included in your medical records. Include all over-the-counter medications and vitamins. If you don't have a list, toss all your pill bottles in a bag and bring them with you to every doctor visit. If you see multiple doctors, update your prescription list with each of them because some may start or stop a medicine, which the others may not find out about if they don't all use the same computerized medical record system. Doctors will depend on you to tell them all the prescriptions you're taking.

Seriously ill patients frequently take ten or more medications, several times a day. My patient Mr. George comes to every ap-pointment with a 3 × 5 note card listing all of his medications by name, dose, and how often and when he takes them. Is it Mr. George's responsibility to keep track of his medications? Or is it his doctors' responsibility? Obviously, we share the responsibil-ity, and it's great that we can work on it together.

Before prescribing any new medication, a doctor is required to check to see what other medications the patient is taking, to avoid harmful interactions. It can be scary to think that someone would prescribe a medication without knowing all the other medications you're taking, but it happens. Things can fall through the cracks. Getting all your medicines at the same pharmacy can be another safeguard to protect you from potentially harmful medication in-teractions because your pharmacist will check your records.

Keeping a list of your medications on your person protects you. If you're in an accident or become suddenly ill, it can pro-vide vital information. It also minimizes the chances of mistakes. Carrying a list of your medications is sharing the responsibility. It's another example of where a good patient-doctor partnership can make for better medical care.

Chart 5.2 below is a list of the daily medications for a person with heart disease.

For "as-needed" medications such as short-acting morphine, keep track of how much you take, when, and what happened since you began taking them (see chart 5.1, p. 114). It's the only way your doctor can know how much pain medication you need.

Write on the medication label or on a separate piece of paper what each of your medicines has been prescribed for. Some pre-scriptions may only say, "Take three times a day" and not specify the conditions for which the drug was prescribed. As on chart 5.2, note what the prescription is for: pain, nausea, blood pres-sure, diabetes, heart failure, or constipation.

MEDICAL RECORDS

Ask for copies of all reports. You—not your doctors, health sys-tems, or hospitals—own your medical records. Having copies of your medical records is especially important if you see doctors in different places who are not on the same medical record system. Take copies of reports with you to your doctor visits. Even if reports are sent to all your doctors, they can be lost or delayed in transit, and when they're held up or not circulated, valuable time can be wasted.

CHART 5.2

Medicine	Dose	Instruction	Morning	Midday	Evening	Bedtime
Simvastatin (cholesterol)	40 mg	Once a day				X
Benazepril (blood pressure)	10 mg	Once a day	X			
Carvedilol (heart failure)	25 mg	Twice a day	X		X	
Aspirin (prevents heart attacks and strokes)	81 mg	Once a day	X			
Furosemide (water pill)	40 mg	Once a day	X			
Morphine long acting (pain)	30 mg	Twice a day	X			X
Morphine short acting (pain)	6 mg	Every 4 hours as needed for pain				
Senna (prevents constipation)	8.6 mg	Twice a day	X			X

Many hospitals have programs that give you direct access to your medical records. Sign up for them. You can get your medical records online through services such as MyChart (for systems that use EPIC as the electronic health record) and the Patient Portal (through the Cerner electronic health record). Specifically, you can access your medical history, including your medications, immunizations, and allergies; print records; receive test results; review your doctor's instructions; and receive important health education information. You can also email your doctor, request appointments, renew prescriptions, and see the record of prior appointments.

You may not be able to understand everything in your medical records unless you've been medically trained. If something in your records scares or upsets you, discuss it with your doctor even if you're afraid of what he or she might say. I believe that in most cases, it's better for patients to be well informed than to be in the dark about their illnesses, and the trend in medicine seems to agree. Until recently, doctors and hospitals were reluctant to make radiology reports available to patients right away. Now most allow patients to see those results as soon as they're ready.

When I order a test that could have unfavorable results, I tell my patients, "The reason I'm checking this is because I'm worried that it might be cancer. I don't think it is, but I'm ordering this test to rule it out." Then, if they look up the result or when I call with it, they won't be completely taken by surprise. However, when the news is bad, it's nearly always surprising.

The temptation to access your test results can be hard to resist, but it can have drawbacks. Since you may be able to see those results as soon as or before your doctor, you could be the first one to get the bad news—or think you've gotten bad news. Since you're not a doctor, you may misread or not understand certain information in your records or results.

Getting unfiltered information without your doctor's input may not be the best route. He or she may have anticipated the results and have a plan. It may be preferable for you to wait for your doctor to contact you. Think carefully before looking up the result of a test that could provide bad news. And if you think you've received bad news, call your doctor right away to learn the whole story.

RX

You are your own best advocate, the person who knows your body best. Keep track of the changes you notice in your body; your notes and observations can provide valuable information. Discuss them with your doctor. Take an active role in your care. Medical care is a partnership between you, your family and friends, and your medical team. Doing your part will make it easier for your medical team to do what it takes to help you get the best care—care that's focused on your unique situation.

chapter six

CONTROLLING SYMPTOMS: PAIN, SHORTNESS OF BREATH, AND NAUSEA

DURING SERIOUS ILLNESS, DISTRESSING SYMPTOMS including pain, shortness of breath, and nausea are common. These, and other symptoms can be triggered by your illness or by treatments such as chemotherapy and surgery. Pain, which can be excruciating and hard to bear, is treatable but not fatal. The same for nausea. Shortness of breath, however, is not only physically distressing but also puts you in mortal fear. As you gasp for air, you may be convinced that you're about to die.

When treating serious illness, controlling symptoms is job number one because you can't focus on anything else when you're aching with severe pain, gasping for air, or consumed by nausea. By itself, your serious illness is bad enough. You don't need distressing symptoms adding to your discomfort and further compromising your quality of life.

The good news is that we have many ways to control your symptoms so you can focus on feeling better and getting on with your life. In this chapter, I'll address some of the most common and distressing symptoms—pain, shortness of breath, and nausea—and their treatment. Since pain is so common and feared, I'll start with it.

PAIN

Pain is a warning. It's a signal to our brains that something is wrong. It's a sign of injury or impending injury. It tells us that we have a wound, a broken bone, or a malfunctioning organ. Pain wakes us up and gets us to pay attention, stop what we're doing, and take action to make it better. When pain is intense, it tells us that the problem is serious and should be promptly addressed.

Pain can dominate your life; it can be the only thing you think about and feel. Everything else can seem unimportant. Pain can distract you, occupy your mind, slow you down, isolate you, and limit what you're able to do. It can affect your clarity, attitude, and perception. No one wants to be in pain. Fortunately, most pain can be managed and controlled.

We all have different tolerances for pain. Pain that barely bothers one person can devastate someone else. Pain also defies measurement; we have no blood tests, monitors, or X-rays that can rate the degree or level of your pain. For example, a study [6.1] found no correlation between MRI findings and back pain. The study included 149 men, and each had an MRI of his lower spine. Each was asked if he had lower back pain. Nearly half of the men who said that they had lower back pain had normal MRIs, and a third who reported having no back pain had abnormal MRIs.

Pain is complex. It's more than just neurologic signals entering the brain. Numerous factors are involved, such as who is experiencing the pain, under what conditions, and how it's interpreted. When my boys were little, if they were playing, having fun, and fell down and scraped a knee, they often popped back up and kept playing. But if they were tired or hungry, that very same fall would result in a big cry that needed a big hug.

Adults are no different. If you think that your back pain is being caused by your cancer, you may feel more intense pain than if you think it is caused by a muscle pull. Often, the diagnosis that your pain is caused by something benign will ease it. Try to understand the cause of your pain. When you find that the cause isn't life-threatening or debilitating, it can ease your distress.

An important rule about pain is that you can't tell how much pain someone is in simply by looking at them. I often hear onlookers say, "He sure doesn't look like he is in pain." The fact is, most chronic pain sufferers—those who have pain for days, weeks, or longer—don't look like they're in pain. Sure, if you're riding a bicycle, fall, and break your arm, it will be obvious that you're in pain. You'll exhibit signs of pain: crying, anguish on your face, and a rapid heart rate. The fact that you're in pain will be unmistakable, but not the degree of your pain.

With chronic pain, the outward signs of pain fade. Since so many factors contribute to how you experience pain, you simply have to believe those who say that they're in pain. The only reliable way to measure pain, and nearly every other symptom, is to ask the person experiencing it.

In medicine, we typically ask patients if they have pain and, if so, to quantify it on one of several scales. The most common scale is the 0 to 10 scale. Virtually everyone who has been to the doctor has been asked to rate his or her pain on this scale. It goes like this, "On a scale of 0 to 10, with 0 being no pain and 10 being the worst imaginable pain, how much pain are you having now?"

Generally, 1 to 3 is considered mild pain, 4 to 6 moderate pain, and 7 to 10 severe pain. I've had patients tell me that their pain is 12. They're telling me that their pain is agonizing, that it's off the charts.

Frequently, I ask patients to compare their current pain to other pain they've experienced—for example, to a toothache, a broken bone, or surgery.

A patient of mine at the San Francisco Veterans Affairs hospital was having intense chest pain that he classified as a 10. When I asked him for a comparison, he told me that when he had served in the army in World War II, he had been captured and tortured. That pain was an 8. Enough said. I got it. His pain was excruciating and required immediate attention.

On our palliative care team, we use a simpler scale that is easier for sick patients. Our scale uses words instead of numbers: *none, mild, moderate,* and *severe.* For young children, we use another scale that features pictures of faces instead of numbers or words.

In some situations, patients can't tell us about their pain. We see dementia patients who can't speak but have obviously painful conditions such as broken bones or pressure sores. Researchers have developed reliable ways to assess pain in patients with dementia so they can get good relief [6.2].

In the ICU, we care for patients who are sedated. They can't tell us about their pain or rate it. In these situations, we assess the degree of their pain by looking for indirect signs such as grimacing and a fast heart rate, and we treat them accordingly.

NEUROPATHIC PAIN

Some pain is caused by damage to the nerves that carry pain signals. No bones were broken, no muscles torn. The only damage is to the nerves, which keep firing pain signals to the brain. This type of pain is called neuropathic pain, or pain caused by nerves, and is extremely distressing and hard to treat. Neuropathic pain also tends to be chronic, and people who incur this type of pain also may not exhibit the outward signs that we associate with pain.

Not only do people with neuropathic and chronic pain not look as if they're in pain, they do everything they can to distract themselves from their pain. They watch TV, listen to music, sleep, or talk with friends and family. But if you ask about their pain, they'll tell you it's a 10. Even doctors and nurses may have trouble believing them. They'll often say, "They don't look like they're in severe pain."

> If you or your loved one has a serious illness and chronic or neuropathic pain, get pain control and make sure that it's enough to relieve your pain. It may take several types of medicines to make it tolerable. Explain that you realize you don't look as if you're in pain because you've endured it for so long. Make it clear that you are trying your best to deal with your pain and to distract yourself from it. Although you're trying to reduce your suffering by focusing your attention elsewhere, your pain is still there.

MANAGEMENT

Pain is bad and pain relief is good. You have a right to have your pain treated. Fortunately, we have an arsenal of effective treatments, including many medications that reduce pain—however, all medicines have their downsides.

Relief for people with pain associated with serious illness often means taking opioid medications. Later in this chapter, I'll discuss opioids in detail, but I want to introduce them now. Opioid medications are related to morphine, are powerful, and have side effects. They are also a blessing for people in pain. Opioids are the reason we can reassure people that we can treat their pain as they near the end of life.

If something less than an opioid pain medication will work or if an alternative therapy will help, use those instead of opioids. Heat, ice, braces, massage, rest, acupuncture, and meditation can work well for pain. Try them. They have no side effects and may provide relief alone or in conjunction with other treatments. Just don't sleep with a heating pad on, because it could burn your skin.

Acetaminophen is an extremely popular pain medicine. It is found in many over-the-counter medications such as Tylenol, Panadol, Aspirin-Free Anacin, and Bayer Select Maximum Strength Headache Pain Relief Formula, and it helps many people. When I recommend acetaminophen to patients, they sometimes look at me like I'm crazy. They came to see the doctor, and he's recommending an over-the-counter pill?

If you haven't taken any other pain medication and your pain is mild or moderate, you might get relief from acetaminophen. It has the fewest side effects of all pain medications. One side effect to be aware of, however, is the potential for serious liver damage from taking too much acetaminophen.

Limit your total daily acetaminophen use. Keep the dosage to no more than 3000 mg a day, or 2000 mg a day if you have liver problems. Many over-the-counter cold and sleep medicines contain acetaminophen, and many opioids are formulated in combination with acetaminophen, so read all medicine labels to avoid taking more acetaminophen than you intend.

Martina came to the ER deeply jaundiced and with pain in her right upper abdomen, where the liver is located. She had a cold, a bad cough, and a broken rib that had occurred when she became dizzy and fell as a result of her illness. Martina had been taking an over-the-counter cold and cough medicine that had 1000 mg of acetaminophen per dose. After she fell, her pain was intense, so she was given codeine pills that contained acetaminophen. She also took additional acetaminophen because she was still in pain.

In the ER, her acetaminophen level was off the charts, and her liver enzymes, a test of liver damage, were so high that they exceeded the upper limits of the laboratory test. Martina was in danger of dying from liver failure. We treated her for an acetaminophen overdose and carefully managed her liver failure. Fortunately, she recovered without needing a liver transplant. Had Martina been warned about acetaminophen, she might have avoided this near-fatal experience.

Non-steroidal anti-inflammatory drugs (NSAIDs) are also very helpful. They're available by prescription and over the counter under names such as ibuprofen, naprosyn, naproxen, and others. NSAIDs reduce inflammation, lower fever, and treat pain. However, they can also cause bleeding in the stomach and kidney damage. Be cautious because you may not notice these side effects until the damage has occurred. Older people and those with serious illness are especially at risk.

If you find that you have to take an NSAID on a regular basis—meaning more than a few times a week—check with your doctor. Find out about medicines that can protect your stomach from bleeding, and consider having your kidney function monitored with blood tests.

SHORTNESS OF BREATH

Shortness of breath is called SOB for good reason. It's frightening; patients who suffer from severe SOB dread it more than they fear pain. Patients who have SOB struggle for air and feel like they are going to die. SOB is a medical emergency.

Pain, even excruciating pain, won't kill you. However, severe SOB is suffocating and makes you fear for your life—and with good reason. You can easily panic, feel extremely anxious, and expend all your energy desperately fighting for breath, which wears you down.

Seriously ill people develop SOB from a number of causes, including pneumonia (infection), pneumothorax (air around the lungs), pulmonary edema (fluid in the lungs), asthma, cancer, and pulmonary embolus (blood clots in the blood vessels that bring blood from the heart to the lungs). SOB can be a sign of a potentially fatal condition. Fortunately, treatments for SOB work well.

When people have SOB, especially in the hospital, the first reflex is to give them oxygen. Oxygen helps SOB patients with low oxygen levels. If your oxygen level is low, supplemental oxygen will help you feel better. But if your oxygen level is normal, oxygen is no more effective than cool, fresh air blowing across your face.

Simply opening a window and breathing fresh air may help—in any situation. Although outside air has no more oxygen than inside air, having cool, moving air blowing across your face can provide relief. Cool, fresh air is cheaper, safer, and more easily accessible than oxygen. It's the first thing you should try. Non-medication approaches including meditation, music therapy, massage, relaxation therapy, and addressing underlying stress and emotional distress may also be effective.

Medicines are available to treat SOB, including those that tar-

> Patients with ongoing SOB tend to limit their activity so they don't feel as short of breath. When their doctors ask them to describe their SOB, they often answer that it's not so bad or that it's just mild. What may be lost is that their SOB may be mild because they spend most of the day in a chair, don't walk more than twenty feet, and don't exert themselves. A simple measure of the intensity of SOB may not fully capture its impact on your life.
>
> Be sure to tell your doctor how much activity you can do before you become short of breath. With treatment, you probably will be able to do much more.

get the anxiety that frequently occurs during attacks. Opioids, the same medicines used to treat pain, are the most effective medicines for managing SOB. Usually, small doses provide relief— much lower doses than are typically prescribed for pain.

> I treated Mr. Carson, a fifty-four-year-old man who had severe interstitial lung disease, a scarring of the lung that made it hard for him to get oxygen. He was so short of breath that even with supplemental oxygen he was bedbound. He had to use a bed-side commode because just walking ten feet to the bathroom made him so short of breath that he thought he would pass out. He rated his SOB moderate when he was sitting.
>
> I recommended a small dose of morphine to ease his condition. The next day, when I asked Mr. Carson how he was feeling, he said he was much better but still rated his SOB as

moderate. How could that be? He explained that when he sat up in bed, he wasn't short of breath, but when he walked to the bathroom, his SOB became moderate. His wife added with a big smile, "But he was able to walk to the bathroom and around the room for the first time in weeks." Being able to walk and use the bathroom was an important accomplishment. It gave him back some dignity and control.

> Some doctors are reluctant to prescribe opioids to patients who are short of breath because opioids can slow your breathing. However, studies have found that opioids are safe, even if you have lung disease.

When SOB is caused by fluid around the lung, medications can reduce it. If they're not effective, a tube can be inserted into your chest to remove fluid. I realize that having a tube stuck in your chest sounds awful, and you sure wouldn't allow it unless you truly needed it, but it can provide welcome relief. If fluid around your lungs quickly builds back up, we leave the tube in so you can leave the hospital and drain the fluid at home.

If you're hospitalized because of severe SOB, you may be intubated. A tube, which is connected to a machine that breathes for you, is inserted into your throat and down into your lungs. Intubation is a temporary treatment for people with lung failure in the hope that their lungs will recover enough to allow them to breathe again on their own.

If your SOB is severe, sedation and intubation can relieve it, but being intubated is quite uncomfortable, and you'll probably be sedated.

If you have severe SOB or are at risk for it, decide whether you wish to be intubated. It's a big decision. Decide now, before you have another attack. In determining whether to be intubated, the crucial question is what intubation will achieve for you? Will it help? Will your lungs recover sufficiently for you to breathe on your own? Will it be worth what you'll have to go through?

When seriously ill patients develop lung failure, it's often a sign that the end of life is quite close. Although intubation may delay the inevitable, it may instead just add to your suffering.

WARNING: Unless you make it clear that you don't want intubation, medical facilities and paramedics will intubate you for lung failure or severe SOB. If you're in the more advanced stages of your illness, intubation may well be something to avoid because it's unlikely that your lungs will recover. Make your wishes known. If you don't want intubation, specify so in your advance medical directives. Tell your doctors, family, and friends. Have it noted on your medical records.

Ask your doctor if you're a potential candidate for developing severe SOB. If so, discuss your treatment options and the chances that intubation will help you. Early in the course of your illness, intubation may help get you through a serious SOB episode. As your illness progresses, it may be less likely to help.

Have an honest discussion with your doctor. If you decide you don't want intubation, discuss how to manage your SOB without it. Near the end of life, opioids and antianxiety medicines provide relief. I address this issue further in chapter 14.

NAUSEA

Nausea has numerous causes. As with pain, nausea is not deadly. However, it's not uncommon for me to hear people say that they'd rather be dead than feel nauseated all the time. Fortunately, many medications and treatments help relieve nausea. In chapter 14, I discuss a serious cause of nausea—obstruction of the bowel—in more detail.

A trick that now seems obvious, but wasn't until a nurse told me about it, is to take your nausea medicine before you eat and then take the rest of your medicines after you've eaten. Taking a handful of pills in the morning can make you feel queasy. So talk with your doctor about how to space your medicines, which could help you avoid triggering nausea.

> With nausea, simple things often help a lot. For example, certain foods and smells can make your condition worse. Keep track of those items and avoid them. In general, hot and cold foods are better than anything lukewarm. Fizzy drinks tend to go down easier. Avoid fatty foods, which can trigger nausea. Try having many small meals, as they tend to work better than fewer larger ones.

OPIOIDS

Many seriously ill people must take opioids for pain relief and to treat SOB. However, the epidemic of opioid abuse currently gripping America has made many of my patients afraid of opioids and reluctant to use them. Opioids have gotten a bad rap. The war on drugs and stories about addiction, overdoses, and deaths from prescription pain medications have fanned those fears and kept many seriously ill patients from using these important pain-relieving tools.

Accidental opioid overdoses are a real and alarming crisis. I don't want to downplay the issue. It's tragic, and efforts to limit the use of opioids for people who aren't seriously ill are absolutely appropriate. However, if you're seriously ill, don't let the war on drugs be a war on you and your pain. Although we must cautiously prescribe and use opioids, seriously ill people shouldn't have to suffer because of bias, unfounded fears, and misunderstanding.

Opioids reduce pain and help patients with serious illness have a better quality of life. When you have less pain, you can do more. Being in pain is stressful, and relieving pain can reduce that stress. It frees the mind to focus on things that are far more important. Since opioids are so feared, maligned, and misunderstood, I want to set the record straight and give you important information about opioids and pain management.

Call them opioids, not narcotics. Let's start with what we should call these medicines. Opioids are frequently referred to as "narcotics." I prefer the nonjudgmental word *opioid* because the word *narcotics* has negative, back-alley connotations. It makes them sound illegal, dangerous, and bad. The word *opioid* is derived from the word *opium*, a product of the poppy plant, from which the first pain medications of this type originated. Opioid is the formal name for all medications, natural and synthetic, that act like morphine.

Opioids can be helpful . . . and harmful. As I wrote in chapter 3, treatments are not intrinsically good or bad, and that includes opioids. All treatments should be judged on whether they help you achieve your goals. Usually, the goal for people in pain is to no longer suffer and to do more. They hope to keep their pain from interfering with their ability to fully live their lives.

For those with serious illness, opioids can be a godsend, but opioids can also ruin lives. Opioid abuse and accidental death from prescription opioids is rampant in the United States and a growing problem worldwide. When I treat patients with serious illness, the opioids I prescribe rarely cause harm. Still, I'm cautious about prescribing them. At the same time, concerns about abuse and accidents, while valid, should not keep doctors from prescribing opioid medications or patients with pain due to serious illness from taking them.

Addiction is rare. Unfounded concerns about opioid addiction abound. They keep people from using opioids responsibly and getting the pain control they deserve. I see many patients with serious illnesses who are afraid to use opioids because they worry that they could become addicted. They picture someone living on the street, stealing to get money for drugs, with needle tracks on their arms from using heroin. That's a powerful and frightening image that none of us wants for our loved ones or ourselves.

The risk of seriously ill patients becoming addicted to opioids is exceedingly low. Let's first define addiction. For our purposes, the simplest definition of addiction and the one I teach my students is "The continued use of a substance [in this case an opioid] despite the harm it is causing." That harm can be physical, psychological, spiritual, social, or financial. People at risk for addiction are those who have had a problem with addiction to drugs or alcohol in the past.

If you have a history of problems with cocaine, methamphetamines, alcohol, opioids, or other drugs, let your doctor know. Together you can monitor your opioid use and make sure you're using them safely. When I prescribe opioids to seriously ill patients who have a history of addiction, I let them know that I'm worried about addiction and warn them that using more opioids than prescribed could create more serious problems. If that occurs, I explain, we will have to deal with those problems separately from, and in addition to, the problems caused by their illness.

If you have never been addicted to a substance, your chances of becoming addicted to prescribed opioids is exceedingly low—less than one in a thousand.

When my grandmother had pain from spinal fractures that didn't respond to NSAIDs, I went with her to her doctor. I had coached her to ask for an opioid prescription to relieve her pain. She asked, and her doctor hemmed and hawed. Finally, he said that he was worried she would become addicted. My eighty-six-year-old Safta addicted? Did he know something I didn't? My grandmother never drank alcohol and never took any medications, let alone street drugs or opioids. I smiled, but I had to butt in. I hadn't expected the doctor's response, though maybe I should have. Together my Safta and I managed to convince her doctor that it was safe and she would not become addicted. For a short time, she took small opioid doses, which were very effective.

Many people confuse addiction with physical dependence, but they differ. Physical dependence occurs when you take a medication regularly, usually at least for a few weeks, and experience symptoms if you suddenly stop taking it. Physical dependence is expected and natural. In fact, it's evidence that you've been taking your medicine regularly. Dependence is not addiction. Physical dependence means that your body has become accustomed to the medication, so when you stop suddenly, your body reacts with withdrawal symptoms.

Stopping opioids suddenly can be very uncomfortable, but it is not life threatening. The symptoms of opioid withdrawal include agitation, getting goose bumps or goose flesh, and diarrhea, which tend to go away in a few days. I know of no good reason to suddenly stop opioids you've been taking regularly for weeks or months. If you need or want to stop, wean yourself off slowly. Ask your doctor to suggest a plan.

The last concept to understand is tolerance. Tolerance is also confused with addiction. Tolerance is the need for more medication over time to achieve the same effect. Tolerance occurs with opioids. About a 20-percent increase in a dosage over a year is consistent with tolerance. In general, when seriously ill patients need increased opioid doses it's because their condition is getting worse and causing more pain. A 20-percent increase in a month would make me worry that a cancer has grown or spread, a new fracture has occurred, or that some other problem has arisen.

Side effects away . . . Opioids definitely can cause side effects. When patients start opioids, they can experience confusion or loopiness. They may get sleepy and have difficulty staying awake. Some find these side effects welcome. For example, sleep is a blessing for those whose pain has kept them awake. Most patients, however, don't like opioid side effects. The good news is that they usually go away after a few days. If dosages are increased, the side effects can come back, but they tend to fade again in a matter of days. If your sleepiness continues, dosages can be decreased or you can take other medications that can help you stay awake. Even strong coffee can help.

Opioids can also slow your breathing. We prescribe opioids to ease shortness of breath. However, many physicians worry that those with serious lung conditions will be harmed, or even die, from taking opioids. The evidence proves otherwise. Even people with chronic lung disease can take opioids safely. Of course, we always start at low dosages and increase them slowly. And SOB, as I've noted, tends to respond to much lower doses than are needed for pain.

Don't let fear, yours or your doctors', keep you from using this valuable tool to control pain and shortness of breath. "Start low and go slow" is the mantra for safely using opioids.

Except constipation. Opioids slow your bowels and lead to constipation, which doesn't go away with time like other opioid side effects. Everyone who takes an opioid should also take medicine to move their bowels. I prescribe senna: it's natural, inexpensive, and available over the counter. I've seen patients who were taking opioids and getting pain relief stop taking them because they became constipated, which was worse for them than their pain. I've also seen patients develop prolonged and painful constipation.

If you take an opioid, make sure your bowels move at least every other day. Senna can be taken up to four times a day. If you haven't had a bowel movement in three days, even with senna, talk to your doctor. A number of treatments prevent and relieve constipation. Many patients find that the tried-and-true remedy of prune juice helps. Avoid fiber. Normally, fiber can help regularity, but when opioids cause constipation, fiber makes it worse.

Allergies to opioids are rare. Opioids seldom cause serious allergy with swelling and/or rashes, but they can. Patients more commonly report that a certain opioid did not sit well with them. Some patients have nausea or can't urinate. Usually, neither of these side effects goes away, and the inability to urinate is a medical emergency.

Vilma's pain was acute and hard to control. We tried one medication after another, hoping to give her relief. A few days after I first examined her, she became delirious. She was confused, kept taking off her clothes, and didn't sleep. Her oncologist asked if it could be the pain medicine. I didn't think so. I had used that medicine hundreds, maybe thousands, of times and never saw a similar reaction.

But as I thought about it further, I realized that the timing was right and it was possible that the opioid was causing her delirium. We stopped Vilma's opioid and put her on a different opioid, at a lower dosage. Within twenty-four hours, she was back to normal and embarrassed. I felt terrible that our medication had had such a profound side effect, but I was glad that we were able to stop it.

> It's impossible to predict how you'll respond to a particular opioid. If, after you start taking an opioid, you have an unpleasant reaction or feel worse, it could be a side effect of the medicine. Most unpleasant side effects are specific to a particular opioid and individual. If you change opioids, side effects tend to resolve and may not recur.

Some people fare better with opioids than others, and some fare better with a particular opioid than others. Opioid receptors vary from person to person. At this time, we don't know how to pair a particular variation of opioid receptor with a specific opioid, so it takes trial and error to make the best match. If the opioid you're taking just doesn't feel right or causes too many side effects, tell your doctor and try another one.

While opioid allergies are rare, when patients are given higher doses, a serious complication known as myoclonus can occur. Myoclonus is involuntary muscle twitching. It can be limited to one part of the body or affect the entire body. It is usually very uncomfortable and distressing. Although myoclonus is usually triggered by high opioid doses, it also can be caused by moderate doses. Reducing the opioid dosage or switching to another opioid usually relieves myoclonus, but if that doesn't help, other medicines can. If you or your loved one develops myoclonus, notify your doctor right away.

The dosage, as a number, is unimportant. I've had patients say to me, "Dr. Pantilat, that's such a big dose of morphine." To which I explain, "The right dose is the one that works for you." Certain opioids, including morphine, oxycodone, hydromorphone, and fentanyl, have no maximum dosage. Patients who have taken those medicines for months or years, or whose intense pain is increasing, may need very high doses.

I tell my patients not to worry about dosage. As long as they're getting pain relief without side effects, the dose is right. We always "start low and go slow." It may take a few days to get the dose right, but starting low and moving forward cautiously is the safest route. I warn my students to avoid the two main dangers when prescribing opioids: (1) giving too much too fast and (2) not giving enough to relieve the patient's pain.

If increasing the dose gives you better pain control, you're moving in the right direction. If more medicine doesn't help, then you might need to switch medicines or try something different.

No opioid is "stronger" than another. All opioids are strong pain relievers, but you'll need different doses of one opioid to get the same amount of pain relief that you get from another opioid. The differences occur because of the pharmacology of the medications, not their inherent ability to relieve pain.

We teach doctors how to compare the dose of one opioid with another to achieve equivalent levels of pain relief. For example, 30 mg of morphine orally may provide the same pain control as 7.5 mg of hydromorphone. This doesn't mean that hydromorphone is better or stronger; it just metabolizes differently. So don't choose one opioid over another because you think it might be stronger. Speak with your doctor to figure out which opioid is best for you.

Methadone is not just for addicts. Methadone is an opioid that is best known as a treatment for heroin addiction. Less known is the fact that it's an effective medicine for people with serious illness and pain. Methadone works like morphine, but it is naturally long acting. Heroin addicts can substitute methadone for heroin because it's much safer for them to use. Methadone prevents the uncomfortable effects of withdrawal from heroin for more than twenty-four hours. It's a convenient, once-a-day medicine to prevent withdrawal symptoms and reduce heroin cravings. Don't let its use for withdrawal keep you from using methadone for pain relief.

While methadone effectively treats withdrawal symptoms for more than twenty-four hours, it only controls pain for about eight hours. As a pain reliever, methadone is typically given three times a day.

Methadone has other advantages. It comes in liquid form, while the other most commonly used long-acting opioids are pills that you cannot crush or chew. That makes methadone preferable for those who have trouble swallowing pills or receive nutrition via tubes. Methadone also relieves pain caused by nerve damage.

The metabolism of methadone is somewhat more complex than the metabolism of other opioids, and many doctors are unfamiliar with it. If your doctor is not comfortable prescribing methadone, and the other opioids haven't reduced your pain, ask for a referral to a pain medicine or palliative care expert who can prescribe methadone. A specialist may also have other ideas on how to treat your pain.

Less pain lets you do more. People frequently worry that if they use opioids for pain relief, they'll become confused zombies who sleep all day. The opposite is true. When used to treat pain, opioids help you be more active and more engaged in life. You can think clearly and focus better than when you were in pain. Uncontrolled pain saps your energy and hijacks your mind. It can keep you from getting out of bed, eating, walking, bathing, and interacting with friends and family. When your pain is controlled, you're able to do more.

You get no points for enduring pain—suffering is just suffering. So many of my patients are afraid of opioids. They worry about becoming addicts or being zoned out. They hear about abuse and overdose and are afraid it will happen to them. In reality, the risk of addiction and abuse, especially in people who have no history of addiction, is trivial.

> When you are seriously ill, the fear of opioids is unrealistic, and avoiding opioids can cause you to experience more pain than necessary. I tell my patients that they get no points for suffering. In some religious traditions, inflicting pain on yourself is a sign of devotion. While that may be a form of religious and spiritual expression, pain caused by cancer, heart disease, or stroke is not religious devotion, it's serious, unrelenting suffering. And in this situation, suffering doesn't produce anything good. Be kind and have compassion for yourself. Use opioids to relieve your pain.

Zero pain may not be possible or necessary. As I've stated, we ask patients to rank their pain on a scale of 0 to 10 or a none/mild/moderate/severe scale. I also ask my patients to tell me their target level. For those with severe pain, or 7 to 10 on the scale, a 0 pain level may not be possible, or the opioid dosage needed to reach 0 may lead to unwanted side effects. Patients with chronic pain may also recognize that just lowering their pain level to 3 to 4 would give them great relief and enable them to do much more.

The goal is to find the right balance between pain control and side effects. Determine what pain level is acceptable for you. Then tell your medical team. If they know that your goal is 3 to 4, not 0, they can help you find the right balance. At some point, you may decide that your goal is 0, that you're tired of being in pain and are willing to accept some side effects, including sleepiness. Frequently, that's the goal of patients at the end of life. They're tired of the pain and want to be rid of it completely. We can usually help them reach their goal.

All serious illnesses cause pain, not just cancer. We tend to associate pain with cancer and for good reason. As cancer grows and spreads to bones and other organs, it can cause pain. Pain is common in patients with advanced cancer. It's also seen in every other serious illness, including heart failure, emphysema, stroke, and dementia. In addition to the illness itself, pain can be caused by side effects of treatments like surgery or catheterizations and conditions like diabetic nerve pain or arthritic joint pain. For example, the site where a pacemaker was placed in a patient's chest may continue to hurt even after the wound has healed. Regardless of the cause or the underlying condition, pain is pain, and it can and should be treated.

Opioids do not reduce all pain. Opioids are effective pain-relief medications, but they may not be effective, or they may only be partially effective, in some situations. First, some pain just won't respond or will only partially respond physiologically to opioids—for example, nerve pain.

Second, pain, as I discussed before, is an interaction between the physical input into the brain and our interpretation of the situation. Opioids are great at inhibiting the pain signals but ineffective at changing our interpretation of the situation. When we're anxious, scared, depressed, or stressed, we may experience more pain, and in those situations pain medicines may not help.

To determine if your pain is responding to opioids, make sure that you're taking enough. If your pain decreases when the dosage increases, that shows that the opioids are working. If not, ask your doctor to prescribe a different pain medication. Since we all respond differently to opioids, you may need a different pain medicine. And if your pain is nerve pain, different classes of medications may be needed. If neither of these strategies works, your pain may not be responsive to opioids. Don't take more opioids unless they reduce your pain.

Opioids are just one tool in the treatment of pain. Regardless of the cause of your pain, try other ways of controlling it, such as meditation, massage, relaxation, listening to music, using hot and cold packs, and getting support from a social worker, chaplain, psychologist, nurse, or doctor. These approaches can work wonders. And they don't need prescriptions and have no side effects.

Also consider what else may be going on in your life. Are you experiencing anxiety, depression, or stress, and if so, what is its effect on you? When you're seriously ill, stress is never far away and anxiety is common. Depression is associated with pain. Depression and pain each make the other worse, and treating one can help with the other. Get help for all issues that are negatively impacting your life.

LONG- AND SHORT-ACTING OPIOIDS

Treat pain promptly, when you first feel it. Pain is easier to treat when it's mild than when it becomes more severe. A fundamental principle of pain management is that it takes less medicine to keep pain away than to relieve it once it's out of control.

If you have pain most or all of the time, taking long-acting pain medicine regularly can help. Long-acting pain medicine remains in your body and works from eight to seventy-two hours, depending on the preparation. Never start with long-acting opioids. Start with short-acting ones—those that last for three to four hours—to determine how much you need and whether you need opioids all the time. Then, if you find that you need pain medicine around the clock, your doctor can convert your short-acting medicine to a long-acting preparation.

Common short-acting opioids include morphine, codeine, hydrocodone, fentanyl, hydromorphone, and oxycodone. They typically work for about three to four hours. Morphine, hydromorphone, fentanyl, and oxycodone also come in slow-release formulations that act for eight to twenty-four hours. Methadone and buprenorphine are naturally long acting.

If you use both long- and short-acting opioids, keep them straight. Have the pharmacist clearly mark which is which on the pill bottles and keep them separate. Long-acting medicines can pack a powerful punch, so try not to mistake them for their short-acting counterparts.

Don't crush, chew, or open long-acting pain pills, tablets, or patches, as you could quickly get their entire dose at once, which can harm you.

With pain medications, it's hard to pinpoint exactly how long the relief will last because it varies from person to person. In my experience, about half of those taking long-acting pain medicines need them more frequently than the instructions suggest. If that's you, let your doctor know. The goal should be for you to have steady and continuous pain relief.

If you're in constant pain and using long-acting pain medications, you probably will have periods when you're in more pain. We call these episodes "breakthrough pain" because the pain breaks through the long-acting medicine (see Figure 6.1). Frequently, these episodes are predictable and are caused by physical exertion or changing a dressing on a wound. You may need to take short-acting pain medicine to relieve breakthrough pain.

FIGURE **6.1**

Achieving consistent pain control

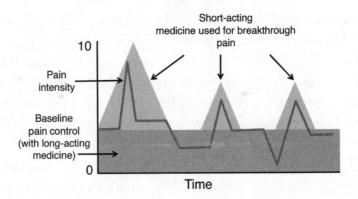

Try to anticipate those episodes and take medication 15 to 30 minutes before they come on so you can control them. You may also have to take short-acting pain medicine for sudden pain that comes out of the blue. Make sure you have short-acting pain medicines at home for such a possibility.

A combination of long- and short-acting pain medications can provide even and steady pain control. If you use only long-acting pain medications and try to treat the breakthrough pain, you may end up taking too much and being sleepy a lot of the time. If you only take short-acting medication, you may always be in pain because the medication may take too long to take effect and may fade too soon.

You'll have good days and bad days with pain and other symptoms. Enjoy the good days, relish them, and take advantage of those times when you have less pain, more energy, or less nausea. On the bad days, take it easy, rest, and listen to your body. You may not need extra pain medicine for every bad day. Often, just slowing down works. However, don't be shy about using pain medicines when you need them so you can feel as well as possible.

CANNABIS

Increasingly, patients are asking about using cannabis to relieve their pain and other symptoms. As we go to press, twenty-three states and the District of Columbia have laws that allow patients to use medical marijuana. (The laws governing cannabis differ from state to state, so know the rules in your area.) Well-designed studies show that cannabis can effectively reduce pain, and many of my patients tell me that it's helped them a lot. For some, it's the only thing that works.

Cannabis can be used in various ways that do not involve smoking or vaporizing it, including consuming it in food or drinks. If you've never used cannabis or have not used it for a long time, be careful! Cannabis can be very potent—more potent than you may remember. It also can have side effects, including making you high, which is why many people use it. As with all pain medications, start low and go slow. Don't mix cannabis and driving. Be smart and safe.

RX

Don't be afraid of opioids. Use them with caution, but use them when your pain is severe. The less pain you're in, the better your quality of life will be. Don't be a martyr. Be kind and compassionate to yourself. When you're in less pain, you'll enjoy life more, and that's what is most important.

chapter seven

HOPE AND THE MOOD ROLLER COASTER

SERIOUS ILLNESS FORCES YOU TO FACE YOUR MORTALITY head on. The future that seemed wide open is now limited. Until you have a serious illness, one that could shorten your life, you don't accept that your time is limited. You ignore that fact, even though you know deep down that it's true.

Learning that you have a serious illness can send you on a mood roller coaster that's filled with countless twists and turns and sudden ups and downs. It can change how you feel physically and make you emotionally vulnerable. Understanding the normal mood changes that accompany serious illness can help normalize it. It also can help you distinguish a bad or sad mood from depression, a disease that requires treatment.

Hope, that essential feature of the human experience, is inexorably tied to mood. It's challenged by serious illness. In the course of my career caring for seriously ill patients, I've come to see hope as one of the most important issues that must be confronted. In this chapter, I want to share what I've learned so that you can understand and deal with hope during your illness.

MOOD SWINGS

Expect to have mood swings that can be intense. Anticipate having good days and bad days, lots of highs and lows. Your mood swings can be sudden, rapid, and extreme. One moment, you may be elated, even euphoric, but moments later or the next day, you may feel down, lower than you've ever been. As a result, your behavior can seem erratic, your judgment compromised, your moods foul, and your attitude poor.

Mood swings are normal; they're part of life. Although many of us have mood swings, they hit seriously ill people harder and more frequently, and are more extreme. During treatment or when you're in the hospital, you might feel especially down. But being discharged and returning home can lift your spirits. A good test result can lift you up, and a bad result can drag you down.

Going through mood swings is disorienting and disturbing. It can wreak havoc on your mind and affect your judgment and behavior, which can frustrate your efforts to lead the best possible life.

When you have mood swings that bring you down, understand that it's OK. Don't beat yourself up. It's reasonable and completely understandable for you to feel blue. Express how you feel to those who care about you. Good friends will want to hear about your sadness as well as your joy. Sharing your emotions eases the burden and lightens your load. It can help you feel better.

When you're down, even during the bleakest times, try to remember that it will get better, things will change, and you'll have ups. Even during the darkest days, some sunlight will break through. So look for those bright spots and embrace them.

Understand that feeling low differs from depression. Seriously ill people will feel low, which is natural and to be expected.

Depression is abnormal, however—even for those who are seriously ill and who are dying. Someone might say, "Well, who wouldn't be depressed in their situation?" While it may be understandable to think that, it's important to realize that not everyone in a bad situation gets depressed. Depression is a disease, a treatable condition that should be promptly addressed even in people near the end of life. Most standard treatments for depression take weeks to work, but some treatments work within days and others that are now being studied could provide relief within hours. Check with your doctor to learn what treatment could be best for you.

Depression taints everything; it darkens your world and makes it worse. It envelops you in a blanket of negativity. Depression impedes your medical treatment because when you're depressed, it's much more difficult to take part in the management of your illness. That makes it harder for doctors and caregivers to help you. When you're depressed, you also can't fight back or help yourself. And worse, depression just plain feels bad.

As seriously ill people get sicker, their decline can make their loved ones, friends, and caregivers depressed. To learn more, see chapter 9, which is devoted to discussing the impact of serious illness on family, friends, and caregivers. Learn to spot depression so it can be promptly treated. Here's the test I use.

Depression test: If you think you or a loved one is depressed, ask the following questions.

1. Are you depressed?
2. Do you still do things that you enjoy?

Believe it or not, question 1, the most obvious question, is extremely important. It gives you a sense of the person's state of mind. If the answer to question 1 is "yes" and the answer to question 2 is "no," it indicates that the person may be depressed.

For many seriously ill people, question 2 may not be that useful, because the reason they no longer do what they enjoy— for example, run, bike, or ski—is due to the physical limitations caused or accelerated by their illness, not the psychological limitation of depression. In these situations, the better question to ask is, "When you think about the future, what do you hope for?"

If people can tell you what they hope for, they're probably not depressed. When they tell you that they can't think of anything to hope for or that they feel hopeless, I worry that they're depressed. Hopelessness is a sign of depression.

> If you feel that you or a loved one is depressed, speak with your doctor and get help. Depression is not a sign of weakness, a moral flaw, or a sign of lack of spirit. Depression is best understood as an imbalance of chemicals in the brain that can be brought on by situations that we face such as serious illness.

Medication restores the balance. I like to think that depression is somewhat akin to diabetes. A simplified explanation of diabetes is that it's due to an imbalance in the response of the body to insulin. Diabetes is not a moral failing, and you can't change how your body responds to insulin with positive thinking. Just as you can't "snap out" of diabetes, you can't just "snap out" of depression.

Depression and diabetes are similar in another way: exercise can help both. Studies [7.1] show that exercise is effective in treating mild depression. Since many people with serious illnesses can't exercise, that's where medications come in. Severe depression is a life-threatening illness and requires medical attention. Don't go it alone—get help for depression from your doctor.

HOPE

Hope is an essential part of the human spirit. Hope is durable; it evolves and persists. It's also a powerful, highly motivating, and driving force. Hope can push you beyond your limits, vault you over obstacles, and thrust you beyond expectations. It can help you keep going when everything seems lost.

Serious illness does not have to destroy your hope. I'm constantly inspired by my seriously ill patients, including those nearing the end of their lives, who tell me about their hopes and then pursue them.

After you've been diagnosed with a serious illness, it may seem impossible for you to hope for anything other than being cured. You may focus all your hope on fighting your disease and beating it. That's understandable. When I speak with patients who have recently learned that they're seriously ill, even those who have an incurable illness, their hope is focused on being cured, on being the person who will beat the odds. Hoping that you'll be cured may be the driving force that gets you out of bed and moves you forward to face another day.

Hoping for a cure doesn't have to be your only hope. Different hopes can coexist. I often tell patients, "Let's hope for the best, but tell me what else you hope for." Frequently, I will simply ask, "When you think about the future, what do you hope for?"

Ask yourself that question. I'm sure that being cured will be your first thought, but what else do you hope for? What about comfort, companionship, dignity, and love? Patients tell me about their other hopes: wanting to be pain-free, be with loved ones, remain at home, visit Machu Picchu, and continue to paint, play bridge, or quilt. Hope is a positive emotion, and thinking about hope in all its positive manifestations feeds our souls.

POSITIVE THINKING

Some patients associate hope with positive thinking and believe that if they think positively, it will help cure their illness. Their positive thoughts, they believe, will help their bodies fight their cancer or rebuild their damaged heart cells. I have no problem with this thinking. Positive emotions such as gratitude, joy, hope, and love support resiliency and brighten moods. Thinking about gratitude every day, finding joy in the simple things in life, and talking about hope are beneficial, not because they cure cancer or heart disease but because they make you feel better.

However, I have concerns. I worry that the idea that positive thinking can cure might be harmful, because if something bad occurs, you might think that it was your fault for not being positive enough. Serious illness is hard enough without feeling that you should have been more positive. During serious illness, guilt and self-blame don't help.

Focusing solely on positive thinking also concerns me because it may lead you to conclude that negative feelings, such as sadness, worry, and grief, are bad and will intensify your illness. Negative emotions are normal responses to serious illness, and we feel better when we can talk about them. I've seen well-meaning families refuse to talk with their loved ones about their worries and grief. "Stay positive," they say. But suppressing sadness doesn't make it go away. Instead, your sadness festers, grows, and isolates you.

I also worry that families that push their loved ones to "stay positive" are giving pep talks to themselves. Talking openly and honestly about our worries, sadness, and grief can foster deep and meaningful connections, which can be extremely beneficial during serious illness.

Grief and sadness arise out of love and gratitude. Hope can be an antidote to sorrow. Find a balance. Talk about all your emotions; it's liberating and cathartic. If you hope to have a meaningful life with deep human connections, expressing your emotions will help you forge stronger bonds.

EVOLUTION OF HOPE

Typically, our hopes evolve. They change with new developments, different states of illness, or simply with time. What we hope for changes and shifts to different levels. Although our hopes change, we continue to hope, but for different things. At least initially, all seriously ill people and their loved ones hope for a cure, to beat the odds.

It's not hard to find stories of people who beat seemingly impossible odds. We've all heard them, and the Internet is full of them. Patients always tell me about an uncle or a cousin who was given six months to live but is still alive and well twenty years later.

Hope for a cure. I encourage it and I join with my patients in that hope. It's always a joy when someone does well and has successful treatment. However, understand that as serious illness evolves, so does hope. You may find yourself setting new goals, hoping for other outcomes that have importance and meaning for you.

Nancy, the mother of my twenty-four-year-old patient Bill, had durable and evolving hope. Bill was in the ICU dying from cancer. At first, I was reluctant to ask Nancy what she hoped for. Her son was dying—what could she possibly hope for other than a cure, which was getting more unlikely every hour and was vanishingly small to begin with. Despite my discomfort, I decided it was important for me to ask.

The first time I asked Nancy, she told me, "I know it's a long shot, but I really hope he beats this cancer." A week later she said, "I just hope Bill can come home." With time, it became clear that Bill was too sick to leave the hospital, and Nancy said, "I hope he can get out of the ICU and into a more private, quiet, and peaceful room for his final days." Unfortunately, that too became impossible. The next day, Nancy told me, "I hope he can be off the machines when he dies. I just want to see his sweet face one more time without all those tubes." As we were preparing to remove the machines and the tubes, I asked Nancy again. She replied, "I hope I can be there, holding his hand, when he dies."

Nancy was with Bill, holding his hand, kissing him, and stroking his face as he died. Nancy never lost hope. Her hope simply evolved, and by understanding what her hopes were, we were able to help her realize them.

The hopes of seriously ill patients tend to evolve similarly. Many reach a point where living as long as possible, regardless of the costs, is not their top priority. It's not even near the top of their list.

Most of the seriously ill people I talk to want to maximize the quality *and* quantity of life. They want to live as well as possible for as long as possible, and that's what we help them achieve. Instead of hoping for a way out, they hope for a way through.

A survey conducted by the California Health Care Foundation [7.2] asked 1,669 adults what issues would be most important to them as they neared the end of life. Living as long as possible was endorsed by only 36 percent, compared to 65 percent who hoped to be comfortable and pain-free, 61 percent who hoped to be at peace spiritually, and 60 percent who hoped that their loved ones would not be burdened by having to make decisions about their care.

EVENTS AND MILESTONES

When seriously ill people have something to live for, it can increase their focus and determination. I've been amazed at how many patients tell me that they want to live long enough to attend a particular event. When they first express their hopes, it can seem unlikely, even impossible, that they could make it, but somehow, some way, they're able to reach their goals. Though I can't prove it, I have no doubt that their wishes help extend their lives.

Often, the hope of a patient with serious illness is to live long enough to attend weddings, bar mitzvahs, confirmations, birthday parties, reunions, births, and other family events. Many do, and accommodations are frequently made. A good example is hospital weddings. I've attended a number of them, some of which were held bedside in the ICU. These events are filled with mixed emotions, contrasts, and incongruities. Let me set the scene.

Marion was a sixty-four-year-old woman with interstitial lung disease, which is a relentless scarring of the lungs. She needed high levels of oxygen just to stay alive. Marion was so sick that she couldn't leave the ICU. When I asked her what she hoped for, she told me that she hoped to see her daughter get married. She explained that her daughter was engaged and the wedding was planned.

"Congratulations," I said. "That's wonderful. When will the wedding be?"

"In ten months, in Napa," Marion replied.

I couldn't imagine Marion being alive in ten months, let alone well enough to leave the hospital or the ICU. So I arranged to speak with Marion and her daughter about the situation and their hopes.

Fast forward a week later to an ICU filled by a bride in a flowing white gown, a tuxedoed groom, identically dressed attendants, and a robed minister. Marion sat propped up in her bed, inhaling oxygen through her nose, and with a corsage pinned to her hospital gown. Our hospital staff, all dressed in different-colored uniforms, gathered in front of Marion's bed, where the ceremony was held. There wasn't a dry eye in the house.

What a beautiful wedding! Marion's wish came true. Because we asked about her hopes, we were able to help her achieve them. Was it what she had imagined? Not at all. But it was joyous, memorable, and meaningful, and the beautiful eclipsed the grotesque. It might not have happened had we not asked about hope.

When I attend hospital weddings, I'm flooded by conflicting emotions: simultaneous joy and sadness and intertwined hope and despair. I'm amazed how rituals about love are performed in cold, antiseptic, and highly technical settings amid electronic noises and alarms. How couples begin their lives together in places filled with sorrow and death.

To me, these hospital weddings are tributes to the human spirit, acknowledgments of the power of hope and love. They show how, in the face of the most hard-to-accept reality, people's strength emerges, how they come together, stand tall, adjust, adapt, make the most of difficult and painful circumstances, and then move on.

Our survival instinct is deeply rooted; it's also massive. We're programmed to fight for our survival. That instinct affects both patients and doctors. It can cause them to lose sight of the fact that mere survival, continuing to live, is not always the best or most realistic objective, especially when the quality of life may be so poor, the suffering so great, and death so inevitable.

Doctors, in their hope to help their patients, may prescribe harsh, aggressive, and even risky treatments. And patients, in their hope to survive, may willingly undergo them.

Often, both doctors and patients misplace their energies. They continue to concentrate on survival and ignore other goals that could still be attained. Too often, the saddest part is that in a vain, and sometimes impossible, attempt to prolong life, they miss out on opportunities to achieve other goals. Those goals may not provide a cure, but they could enhance life by easing the ordeal of serious illness and creating meaningful and memorable experiences.

Leslie, a previously healthy sixty-two-year-old woman, came to the hospital because of shortness of breath that had become so severe that she couldn't walk more than a few steps without getting winded. Tests revealed that she had mesothelioma, a serious, highly aggressive cancer in her chest, surrounding her lungs. She wasn't prepared for the diagnosis, and it came as a jarring shock.

We consulted an oncologist, who explained Leslie's treatment options to her. Leslie asked a lot of questions and understood that her treatment could extend her life but that it wouldn't cure her cancer. When I asked Leslie what she hoped for, her response was like Marion's.

"I just want to make it to my son's wedding."

"When is the wedding scheduled?" I asked.

"In a year."

"Any chance he could get married sooner?" I asked, and explained that she would be fortunate to live another year.

Shortly after our conversation, the wedding was moved up to the following month. Leslie waited to start chemo until after the wedding because she was worried that the treatment might make her too sick. The oncologist had assured Leslie that she could wait.

Leslie attended the wedding, but she had complications and had to return to the hospital. When I visited her, she was making a quilt.

"Who is that for?" I inquired.

"For my grandchild."

"How lovely. When is the child due?"

"I don't know. My daughter-in-law isn't pregnant yet. But she will be."

Leslie was making the quilt for a grandchild she would never meet or get to know. Completing that quilt was her motivation, her focus, and her hope. With great determination, Leslie worked diligently on the quilt, finished it, and died peacefully five months after her initial diagnosis.

DOWNSIDES OF HOPE

Although hope is a great motivator that can keep you moving forward, it can also cause harm. Hope can alter your judgment, divert you, make you act rashly, and cause you to reject
sound advice. It can blind you to what others can plainly see.
When you're seriously ill, it's natural to hope for a cure, but a
cure may not be possible. If you focus all your time and energy
on being cured, it can keep you from taking care of other important business, making crucial decisions, and accomplishing
achievable goals. You may spend all your time chasing a cure,
seeking multiple options, and trying experimental treatments.
The pursuit of a cure can undermine the very reason you want
a cure: to have more time with loved ones. In the end, you lose
out on both.

Pursuing a cure may not only distract you from the present,
but it can also expose you to other, and even greater, dangers.
For instance, the operation for the left ventricular assist device or
the next round of chemo may cause more harm than your disease
itself. It may hurt more than help. You can have a bad reaction,
experience side effects, feel awful, and land in the hospital. Although you'll still be alive, you'll have no life.

In order to live better and longer, your best course of action
may be not to pursue disease-directed treatment. Now, I know
that sounds counterintuitive because most of us instinctively
think that we have to do everything possible to eliminate our
illness. However, I've seen too many patients continue taking
treatments that didn't help and even became harmful. They felt
that they "had to do something."

The trouble is that the treatments may not work; they may not
cure your illness. Plus, they can make you sicker. Avoiding those
treatments can conserve your energy, strengthen your body, and

enhance its ability to get through your illness. Thich Nhat Hanh, a Vietnamese Buddhist teacher, said, "Don't just do something, sit there." I often think of this saying when I'm speaking with seriously ill patients who are contemplating trying potentially toxic interventions that are not likely to help them.

Unfortunately, doctors often contribute to the downsides of hope. Doctors may think that:

(1) They can *give* their patients hope by telling them that they can cure their illness.

(2) If they tell their patients that their illness is incurable, they'll destroy hope.

Although hearing that no cure exists is hard to take, it will help you focus on what you can actually accomplish. It can also force you to refocus, adjust, and reexamine your goals.

Push your doctor to explain exactly what's possible. If she seems hesitant or reluctant, explain that it's important to you that she be honest. Make it clear that you would like to get enough information to understand where you truly stand so you can make the best decisions.

Periodically, ask yourself what you hope for, what's most important to you at this time. Then see if a particular treatment will help you achieve what you hope for and whether it will do more good than harm. If you decide to undergo a treatment, go in with your eyes open and knowing the risks.

FALSE HOPE

No discussion about hope can be complete unless it considers false hope. You may ask, "What's the harm in hoping for a cure? Why not let people believe that a cure is possible until the end? Why not let them think that they're not dying even when they are?"

Before I answer, I want to point out that every seriously ill patient I've cared for was aware that they were seriously ill. They may not have wanted to discuss it, but they knew. As you get weaker and lose your appetite, as people speak in hushed tones outside your room, as you go to the doctors' office or the hospital more frequently, you know the score. You realize that something is going on and it's bad.

My concern is that false hope—hope that's not reality based—can be worse than no hope at all. It can make you squander your time, energy, and resources, and it can send you off in a wrong direction. It can cause you to delude yourself, be unrealistic, and make poor decisions. False hope is no hope at all.

Sergey was an eighty-year-old man who was originally from Lithuania. His wife, Yelena, who was a few years younger, had advanced dementia. She had suffered many infections and complications that left her a shell of her former self.

When Sergey brought Yelena to the hospital, she was unable to communicate and was receiving nutrition through a tube. It was clear that further treatments couldn't help Yelena get better. I encouraged Sergey to focus on Yelena's comfort. I also asked him what he hoped for. "I hope she gets better, wakes up, and is her old self again," Sergey said.

I didn't see any way that Yelena would recover, so I tried to explain that, while I could sympathize with his hope, I couldn't see any path to it. "Doctor, you don't understand," Sergey insisted. "Where there's life, there's hope. When I was young, I served in the Soviet army during World War II. I fought in the Battle of Stalingrad, where thousands of people died of starvation. We had no food, but I never lost hope. I ate scraps, frozen potato peels, and scavenged for anything to eat. I didn't give up, I never lost hope, and I survived."

I realized that as horrible as Sergey's odds had been in Stalingrad, they were better than Yelena's odds of recovering. I also understood the source of Sergey's hope and his iron-willed determination, and I knew his position was firm. To him the miraculous had happened once before, and it could happen again—if he didn't lose hope. So I told him that I understood. I think that Sergey couldn't face a future without his wife. They had been married for sixty years and had been through so much together. We tried to address that sadness, but we couldn't help Sergey find a way through.

We discharged Yelena, allowed her to go home, and arranged for home care for her and Sergey. As much as I dislike false hope, I understood the depth of Sergey's hope and his need to fight for survival.

Addressing false hope is difficult. No one wants to destroy someone's dreams. When I hear patients express false hope, I'm always thrown because I know that I'll have to deliver bad news. I don't know of a good way to keep them from being let down. I try to gently explain, to softly set them straight, but it doesn't always work. So I say, "I wish it were the case that we were looking at four or five years, but unfortunately, I think we're looking at something more like months."

I choose my words carefully and try to be direct and realistic. I understand how deeply my words will hurt, so I try to be kind and compassionate and do what my experience has proven is best. A realistic picture keeps patients from wasting their time. Does it take away one type of hope? Yes. Does it help them focus on what's most important? Also yes. They can assess how they think about their lives, how they want to spend their remaining time, and what they can still hope for.

RX

I often think about what I would hope for and what I would do if I knew that I only had a year to live. I'm sure I would change some things. I'd work less and plan for succession at work. I would spend more time with my wife, children, and close friends. I would travel to places on my bucket list.

I'd also stop flossing. Yes, that sounds trivial, but I hate flossing. The only reason I floss is because I hope to have my teeth for another fifty years. But if I had only one year left, I'd stop flossing today.

When you look to the future, what do you hope for?

When you think about what lies ahead, what worries you the most? What are you doing about it?

We all have hope. Talk about your hope, cultivate it, and share it.

chapter eight

CAREGIVING AND SUPPORT

Serious illness affects those who are ill and also impacts their family and friends. These loved ones not only witness serious illness, but they may also participate in it as caregivers. In the course of serious illness, caregiving by family and friends is the norm.

During serious illness, patients' families and friends grieve. Watching their loved ones suffer and seeing their health decline is heartbreaking and can damage their own health. And when family and friends are their loved ones' caregivers, the effect on them can be even greater. Caregiving takes an emotional and physical toll, but it can also be tremendously rewarding. It can be as great a gift to the caregiver as it is to the patient receiving care.

Caring for seriously ill people can also be thankless. Patients can be demanding, difficult, and unrealistic. They may have unreasonable hopes, standards, and beliefs. Deep down, they may hope that their caregivers will be miracle workers, and when reality intrudes, they may take their frustrations out on their caregivers.

In serious illness, caregiving by family and friends is nearly universal. Often, professional caregivers are also needed to help during these difficult, gut-wrenching times. By "professional caregivers," I mean people who are paid and tend to be strangers. Some professional caregivers have advanced health-care degrees—for example, nurses and therapists—but most do not.

Patients who want, but can't afford, professional care may feel embarrassed that their family or friends have to care for them. They may feel that it's akin to accepting charity. They may also be afraid that the care they receive from their family and friends won't be as good as the professional care that they can't afford. Their feelings can create hurdles that their family and friends as caregivers must overcome.

Two basic caregiver categories exist: (1) family and friends and (2) professionals. In this chapter, when I refer to caregivers, I'm referring to people in both groups who provide care in patients' homes, not in health facilities. First, I'll look at category 1: family and friends. I'll highlight some of the challenges and rewards of caregiving and provide specific suggestions to ease the job of caregiving for everyone involved. Next, I'll cover professional caregivers and discuss the critical role they play in helping patients get good care at home.

CAREGIVING AND HOME HEALTH CARE

I first want to distinguish caregiving from specific health care services that are provided in the home and called home health care. Home health care is a distinct insurance benefit for specific health episodes and medical tasks. Home health care is intended for people who are homebound and need skilled medical services that can include nursing care for managing wounds, IV medications, social work, physical therapy, occupational therapy, and speech therapy. Home health care is provided only for a limited time. When the medical need—for example, for wound care—is met, home health care for that episode will end.

Although home health care is provided at patients' homes, it's not the type of caregiving I'll address in this chapter. The caregiving I'll cover helps patients with their daily activities like bathing, cooking, eating, dressing, shopping, toileting, and companionship. The home health care benefit doesn't include these activities. The caregiving I will discuss also often helps with medical activities such as giving medicines including IVs, helping with exercises, and recording symptoms and vital signs.

FAMILY AND FRIENDS CAREGIVING

Caregiving is hard and demanding. It can become a full-time job with a heavy workload, and the working conditions can be challenging. Caregiving is physically and emotionally punishing. It can take a heavy toll on caregivers' health, which tends to surprise them. As their patients'/loved ones' illness continues and intensifies, the effect on caregivers sneaks up on them. Family members and friends often have to reduce their work hours or quit their jobs because it becomes too much for them, which can create additional financial burdens.

Family members and friends take caregiving seriously. Many do it willingly. They roll up their sleeves and jump right in. They consider caregiving a privilege and find it rewarding. Some are natural caregivers. Taking care of others is their passion, what they feel they were born to do. They take to caregiving enthusiastically and usually provide excellent care.

But caregiving isn't for everyone. Some people simply are not cut out to care for others. It's not in their nature, and it makes them nervous, anxious, and ill at ease. They may not have the patience, confidence, or knowledge needed to be a good caregiver or want the responsibility. Some may not be up to it physically, emotionally, or because of other demands.

Those who don't volunteer to care for close family members or friends often feel guilty. They think that it's expected of them and by not pitching in, they're shirking their responsibility and letting their family and friends down. However, since everyone isn't suited to giving care, they shouldn't punish themselves. Plus, taking on tasks that one can't perform well can be harmful to both the patients and the reluctant caregivers. These friends and family members can help in other ways: by shopping, cooking, running errands, or simply being available to hang out with the patient and enabling caregivers to get some time to rest.

Family members and friends often fear that they're not sufficiently prepared to be caregivers. When they give care, they tend to worry that they're not doing a good job or not doing enough. They also worry that they're not making the right decisions and that they may make mistakes and harm their loved ones. In my experience, family caregivers are extremely diligent and provide superb care. Their worries are overblown and seldom pan out. If you have these concerns, speak to health care professionals. Nurses and hospice workers can be outstanding teachers and advisors.

Most basic caregiving tasks can be learned. They don't require extensive medical training. Family members and friends can quickly learn to use feeding tubes, inject blood thinners or insulin, give pain medications, and perform many other duties. Although these and other tasks are technical, lay people routinely learn to perform them expertly.

In the previous chapter, I described how serious illness can be an emotional roller coaster: how patients' feelings can fluctuate from extreme to extreme. Caregivers frequently take the same ride. As their loved ones get sicker, caregivers invariably wear down. They worry and grieve. They often become exasperated, irritable, tired, and short tempered. Watching loved ones suffer and fight valiantly, only to get weaker, is emotionally shattering; it drags caregivers down. It can batter their emotions and devastate their health.

Most caregivers try to control their emotions. They try to be pleasant and to put on a brave, happy face, but since they're only human, their frustration and pent-up feelings invariably surface. In spite of their efforts to control their emotions, they may respond sharply, abruptly, dismissively, and even cruelly. They feel horrible about their outbursts and know that their reactions sting, which makes them feel even more ashamed. They hate the fact that they treated their loved ones so callously.

These reactions are understandable. In fact, they're absolutely normal. They're the same feelings parents have when their infant keeps them awake night after night: of course they love their child and want to comfort him, but they're also exhausted, frustrated, and sleep deprived. The caregivers are on edge, plagued by mixed emotions, shame, and guilt, and they wish that they had not reacted so impulsively.

Caregiving is no different than any close relationship, which is to say that we often take liberties with those we love and treat them in ways that we wouldn't treat others. Serious illness and the stress it causes do not turn us into saints. If anything, the difficulties and challenges inherent in close relationships are magnified by serious illness. It helps to take breaks, take deep breaths, and count to three before responding and to be understanding, tolerant, and forgiving. Fortunately, our closest loved ones are also those who are most likely to forgive our shortcomings and outbursts.

> Being a caregiver can be particularly intense for spouses. Day after day, they're with their partners, witnessing their ups and downs, sharing their hopes and disappointments, watching them suffer and seeing them fade. Frequently, they don't get breaks. And since many spouses, like patients, are older, the rigors of caregiving can be even more difficult for them.
>
> Many spouses also have to deal with pressing financial problems. In addition to the costs of their spouse's medical care, both they and their spouse may not be working, so less income may be coming in.

Serious illness and caregiving is a marathon; it's a long, grueling test. Since caregiving can be so stressful, care for the caregiver is critical. I can't emphasize enough that breaks are critical. Caregivers frequently don't take them often enough. Hospice services can provide respites for a few hours or a few days. Even a few hours can make a huge difference.

Mrs. Chang, an eighty-one-year-old with dementia, was admitted to the hospital after passing out. She was found to have pneumonia and an abnormally slow heart rhythm that caused her to lose consciousness and fall. She needed a pacemaker, but first we had to treat her pneumonia.

Mrs. Chang had seven children. Every morning on rounds, we would meet one of them who had taken his or her turn spending the night with her. Later that morning, another would come to take the day shift. For the nine days Mrs. Chang was hospitalized, one of her children was always with her.

Most patients don't have those resources. They don't have seven children who can take turns being with them. However, their family and friends can team up, rotate, and take caregiving shifts.

> When people with dementia, even mild dementia, are hospitalized, they can become disoriented, particularly at night. They can also get agitated and be at high risk for complications such as falls. An effective strategy to reduce that risk is having someone familiar be with them, especially at night when they're more likely to become agitated. It's important to reassure them that everything is OK and help keep them calm. Mrs. Chang's children recognized the importance of having someone familiar stay with their mother during her hospitalization.

Seriously ill patients worry that they will burden their family and friends. For many patients, it's an obsession. The constant fear that they may become physically, emotionally, and financially dependent can affect their attitudes and their health. It can complicate their treatment, slow their recovery, and make it more difficult for them to get through their illness. Typically, family and friends don't share the fear that the patients will become a burden.

PROFESSIONAL CAREGIVERS

Hiring a professional caregiver allows the family to be the family and the friends to be the friends. However, when professional caregivers are on board, family and friends typically still provide some care. Since they don't have to provide all the care, family and friends can spend time with patients doing other things—things they both enjoy. Spending non-caregiving time with their loved ones also gives family members and friends great satisfaction and cherished memories.

Professional caregivers know the ropes. They're experienced, have cared for other patients, and have been through similar situations before. Most are honest and reliable, have good bedside manners, are not intrusive, and are adept at handling sticky situations and emergencies.

Professional caregivers rarely have the same emotional attachment to patients as the patients' family and friends. For the most part, they're strangers who have come in to do difficult jobs. But most professional caregivers are truly caring and provide quality care, and frequently they form close personal bonds with patients and patients' families. And because most caregivers have experience providing care to seriously ill people, they can provide reassurance and be a calming presence.

> I am a big fan of professional caregivers. Even when family and friends want to provide most of the care, adding a professional caregiver to the mix allows everyone to have a break and provides a more objective individual to help out. Hiring a professional caregiver is not a failure on the part of the patients' family and friends; it's recognizing what is best all around.

The best way to find a caregiver is by asking your medical team, family, and friends. When they've had good experiences, they'll give you referrals. If they can't, widen your search within your community. Focus on finding experienced caregivers who understand your situation. When you contact them, explain what you think you need.

When my mom came home from the hospital after being diagnosed with lung cancer, she resisted having professional caregivers. She wanted only my aunt Ayala, her sister, to care for her. At first, when my mom was still able to get out of bed by herself, it worked. Then one night she fell as she was on her way to the bathroom and couldn't get up. My aunt tried but couldn't get her back into bed.

After her long night of struggle, my mom agreed to have more help. My sister knew of someone who had been a caregiver for a family friend. They contacted Libby, who came to meet my mom. They hit it off. Libby moved into my mom's home and, along with my aunt, provided all her care. Libby quickly became a member of the family and was with my mom until she died. Libby then cared for my sister's mother-in-law and later for my father-in-law. Finding Libby was a godsend! It was a great comfort to know that our loved ones were in good, caring, and compassionate hands.

Many patients and their families are concerned about the cost of caregiving; they're afraid that they can't afford it. Employing a professional caregiver is often not as expensive as you might think. Caregivers usually offer various types and levels of service that enable you to come to an arrangement that will work for you. Also, you won't necessarily need 24/7 help. Often, just a few hours a day can make a big difference. Most people don't need nurses, but rather a caring individual who can attend to their basic needs. And most caregivers can be taught, just like family caregivers, how to give medications, how to handle tubes and drains, and how to record patients' symptoms and responses to treatment. Contact both freelancers and agencies to learn what they offer and charge. What you find may surprise you.

AGENCY OR FREELANCE?

You can hire professional caregivers on your own or through agencies. Hiring freelancers may be cheaper and may give you more control, but it takes more work.

Agencies offer the advantage of prescreening caregivers and usually can provide a caregiver on short notice. If you're in the hospital, leaving tomorrow, and need a caregiver, an agency may be your only option. Agencies can also provide replacements if your usual caregiver is ill or is otherwise unavailable.

Agencies can provide caregivers who have different skill sets and levels of training. However, agencies also have rules as to what caregivers can and cannot do and will not let their caregivers perform certain tasks, especially those that they're not trained in. (Ironically, family caregivers are often put in positions of taking on tasks without formal training.)

A caregiver's role can vary over time. It can range from simply being a companion to virtually being a nurse. Before you start the hiring process, list all the tasks you want the caregiver to perform. Review the following categories and try to identify, as specifically as possible, the tasks to be performed. They can include:

> › Personal care: bathing, shampooing, toileting (using bedpans, commodes, diapers), grooming, and dressing.
> › Movement: transportation to appointments and activities; assistance with walking, lifting, physical exercises, and getting into and out of bed; transfer to wheelchairs; and help with wheelchairs and walkers.

> Meal preparation, serving, and cleaning up.
> Taking and recording vital signs, other symptoms, and responses to treatment.
> Turning and positioning bedbound patients, massaging, and facilitating stretching and range-of-motion exercises.
> Assisting with and giving medication.
> Household tasks: changing linens, washing dishes, doing laundry, dusting, cleaning floors and furniture, shopping, and emptying trash.

Before you start the hiring process, know what you want and how many hours each day caregiving will be required and at what times. Identify all your needs and write them out. Also outline the care needed during a typical day from the time you wake up until you go to sleep. Think about whether you need someone during the day, at night, or both.

Be sure to list the times when you eat, nap, take medication, exercise, and do other activities. Specify any dietary needs and restrictions—for example, heart failure patients often need to limit how much they drink each day. If you need a caregiver with you more than eight hours a day and more than five days a week, you will need more than one caregiver. Even professional caregivers need rest and time away.

Caregiving is stressful work, and it doesn't serve anyone if caregivers get burned out. No one can be expected to work twenty-four hours a day, seven days a week—even though many family caregivers do just that. Tired workers lose focus and make more mistakes, so make sure your caregivers are rested, fresh, and alert.

FREELANCE CAREGIVERS

To hire a freelancer, contact applicants and have them fill out applications and give references. You can post the job on Internet job sites, on neighborhood forums, and through your network of family and friends. Then screen applications, talk with applicants by phone, and check references. Invite those you like and who seem like a good fit to interview, and, for the ones you like the most, do a background check. During interviews, carefully discuss their duties, what the job will entail, and their previous experience.

Ask them the following:

> How long have you been doing this kind of work?
> Why do you do this kind of work?
> What do you like best about caregiving?
> What do you like least about caregiving?
> What kinds of tasks do you enjoy?
> Who have you worked with? Can you describe your experiences?
> May I contact your references? *Checking references is a must!*
> What specific tasks have you performed/can you perform?
> What tasks are you unwilling to do?
> Do you have transportation to get to and from work and to take me to doctor appointments and/or therapy?
> How would you cover your shift if you were ill?
> What would you do in case of emergency?

Remember, when you hire a caregiver, you're inviting someone into your home to be with you many hours a day. You have to like that person and feel comfortable with him or her. Your personalities need to jive. If you are quiet and don't like to talk much, don't hire a chatterbox. If you like to discuss the news, hire someone who is also engaged in current events. Monitor your caregiver's performance, and if you're not satisfied, cut ties and hire someone else.

At times, caregiving requires a team.

When Doris was getting weaker from cancer, she was adamant about remaining at home. She realized she needed professional caregivers to make this possible. Though her family asked many friends for names of caregivers, they didn't have any leads, so they placed an ad on Craigslist.

The first day, Doris received over fifty responses. She interviewed seven, checked references for five, and hired four to provide seven-day-a-week caregiving. As she got sicker, Doris decided to add a caregiver at night, so one of her caregiver's cousins joined the team. The team of caregivers provided wonderful support for Doris. Some became close friends and were a great comfort to her family. Best of all, they made it possible for Doris to be at home.

You can determine the amount of coverage you want and create your own team. With freelancers, you can hire caregivers with different skills to ensure that you get the range of skills you want and need. Many freelance caregivers are willing to learn and eager to gain more skills.

AGENCIES

Agencies should be state and locally licensed, bonded, and insured. Their caregivers should have good references, have passed drug screenings, and be bonded, insured, and immunized for communicable disease. Agencies should have conducted, and provide you with proof of, background checks on all caregivers' credit, criminal, and driving records.

> Sadly, among all the developed countries, the United States is the only nation that spends more on health care than on social services such as caregiving. I've seen patients who could not afford a caregiver be forced to go to nursing homes, which costs their insurers, often Medicare or Medicaid, far more than what a caregiver would have cost. What a waste! This policy is shortsighted at every level. It's terrible for patients, terrible for families, terrible for insurers, and terrible for society.
>
> Make life better for those with serious illnesses and their families: contact your legislators and tell them to enact changes so Medicare and Medicaid will pay for home caregiving. It would make a huge difference in patients' quality of life.

Most agencies train their caregivers, so they usually perform their duties well. Agencies also handle administrative tasks such as billing Medicare, Medicaid, and insurance companies for you when applicable, though typically caregiving is not covered as a medical benefit.

To find out if you're eligible for financial assistance with in-home caregiving, check your policy; speak with a social worker at your hospital, your doctor's office, or your city or county; or call your insurance company. Some long-term-care insurance covers in-home caregiving. In some situations, assistance programs will compensate family members for being caregivers. These services may vary from state to state and even from county to county. Inquire locally.

If you're thinking about going through an agency, consider asking the questions on the checklist that follows.

Agency checklist:

___ How do you determine what level of caregiving I need?

___ Can I meet prospective caregivers in advance?

___ Do you have consistent assignments, or will the caregivers change on a regular basis?

___ What happens if my usual caregiver is sick or on vacation? Will you automatically send a replacement?

___ What happens if my usual caregiver leaves the agency?

___ How do you handle conflicts between a caregiver and a client?

___ Am I expected to provide meals for the caregiver?

___ What else am I expected to provide?

___ Can your employees drive me/my loved one to appointments or social outings and, if so, are there any mileage charges?

___ Can I talk to former and current clients?

___ How much is your hourly rate? (Rates vary with agencies, training levels, and experience.)

___ What other charges or fees may I be asked to pay?

___ Do you accept Medicare and Medicaid payments? And will they pay for any caregiving?

___ Do you accept payment from _____ (your insurance company's name)?

___ Do you offer a payment plan or other types of financial assistance?

___ Do you accept credit cards?

___ Are your caregivers employees or independent contractors?

___ Will you take care of all payroll paperwork (including taxes, insurance, and benefits), or will that be my responsibility?

CAREGIVING AT HOME

Family caregiving tends to evolve slowly over time. At first, it may just entail helping patients take medicine, get up and down stairs, or dress. It may initially be only for a few days after chemotherapy or a week or two after surgery. Slowly, it may evolve to providing help with more needs more often.

When caregiving evolves slowly, it may be difficult to decide when to get more help, because one day is usually not much different than another. Changes can be subtle, easy to miss. Be alert. Try to get more help before the caregiver gets tired, overwhelmed, or burned out.

Caregiving can also become a necessity in one fell swoop—for instance, after a stroke. When it does, families may be overwhelmed. They may be nervous and afraid that they can't do the job. Some may be unable to take time away from their jobs because they need the money to keep the family afloat. Patients may be in shock. They may be the main breadwinners and under great financial stress.

When a professional caregiver first arrives at a patient's home, the atmosphere can be bleak. Patients and their families have been going through turmoil, and the fact that they now need caregiving can make them sadder, more fearful, and more difficult. Many patients and their families are uncomfortable, even distrustful, of having strangers in their homes. It's hard for them to get used to caregivers sleeping, eating, and constantly being there, and they frequently get in each other's way. The atmosphere for caregivers can be awkward, chilly, and even hostile—at least initially.

On the other hand, the arrival of a competent, compassionate, and kind caregiver can be like the cavalry coming to save the day. Caregivers can provide a huge sense of relief. Calm can be restored and confidence built as caregivers get to work. Many caregivers fit right in and become trusted and indispensable members of the household.

Your home is probably not set up for caregiving and may need to be rearranged. You may have to be moved to another floor or to a different room. Special furniture, equipment, and supplies may have to be brought in and placed where they're most easily accessible. Equipment can include hospital beds, oxygen tanks, suction machines, bedside commodes, and IV poles and pumps.

When my grandparents were looking for an apartment in Denver, my grandmother really wanted two bathrooms: one for her and my grandfather and one for guests. My grandfather, being a very practical and frugal individual, thought they would be fine with just one bathroom. My grandfather won. As he got sicker with lung cancer, he got too weak to get up to use their bathroom. Hospice brought in a bedside commode. As they placed it near his bed, he looked at my grandmother with a smile and said, "Well, Manya, now we have the two bathrooms you always wanted."

Rearrangements may be difficult to make and hard for families to live with. However, they can also be beneficial for patients as well as their caregivers.

When Evelyn was receiving care at home for a rare cancer, she had difficulty getting out of bed, which made it harder for her caregivers. It also isolated her upstairs in her bedroom. So her family rearranged her home to make it easier for her, as well as for her friends and caregivers. They moved Evelyn from her upstairs bedroom to the first floor, in the dining room, which was adjacent to the kitchen; they set up a hospital bed and a large-screen TV and placed some chairs around her bed. Then, when visitors came, they didn't have to go upstairs to the bedroom and had places to comfortably sit by Evelyn's bedside. Since the dining room was next door to the kitchen, which was a hub of activity, Evelyn could be part of all the goings on. When she needed privacy, visitors were able to easily slip away into another room, putting them more at ease because they didn't feel that they were intruding on Evelyn's space. Rearranging her home created a comfortable environment for Evelyn, her caregivers, and her visitors to spend time together in a more relaxed way.

THE TASKS OF CAREGIVING

When caregivers begin caring for you, stress that you want them to be honest with you despite how they think you might react. Make it clear that you want them to tell you what they think and what they can and cannot do. Caregivers can provide valuable information. They can make observations and have insights and understandings that you would miss. But remember, caregivers typically are not medical professionals, so take any medical recommendations with a grain of salt or two.

Caregivers are often asked to do a lot, which can make them feel overwhelmed and under great pressure to get it all right. They also worry about making mistakes that could harm the patient. It's vitally important that both family and professional caregivers feel comfortable regarding the duties they have to perform.

Tell your caregivers to let you know if they're uncomfortable about performing any duties. Explain that you don't want them to agree to take on tasks under pressure and then find that they can't give an injection or pack a wound. It's essential for you and your family to know what your caregiver feels he or she can do competently, what they can't do, what they're willing to learn, and what they are not.

Some of the usual tasks that caregivers may have to perform include arranging and coordinating patients' appointments and treatments; managing medications, IVs, and feeding tubes; giving injections; keeping detailed records; providing updates and progress reports; lifting, turning, and moving patients and equipment; cleaning, bathing, and changing patients and their dressings; taking care of their toileting needs; cooking, cleaning, and shopping for them; and doing their laundry. The pressure on caregivers to perform well can be intense.

Caregivers should keep good records on the care they provide and the patients' responses. They're the eyes and ears of the doctors and nurses. The information they record helps doctors and nurses understand how patients are responding to treatments and progressing. Refer to chapter 5 on managing your medical care for a discussion of how to monitor symptoms.

Make sure that your caregivers know your preferences for care and especially for end-of-life care. Those preferences should also be completely clear to your family and medical team. No doubt should exist as to whether you want the paramedics called if you have trouble breathing or if you want CPR or to go to the hospital. Not only do you need to have these discussions with your caregivers and family, you must be sure that they will respect your wishes.

SPECIFIC CHALLENGES

Some patients are resistant. They may not want caregivers in their home, invading their terrain. Accepting care, they may reason, is an admission that they're seriously ill, which they may not be ready to concede. They figure, "If my husband is able to take care of me, I must not be that sick." So they make hiring a caregiver more difficult by finding fault with every applicant, rejecting them, and not cooperating with those who are hired. In my experience, patients who initially fight the idea of bringing in caregivers come around, and their objections usually quickly pass. Caregivers tend to become a part of the family and forge close, caring relationships with their patients and patients' families.

Dementia (Alzheimer's disease) and degenerative neurologic conditions such as ALS (amyotrophic lateral sclerosis, or Lou Gehrig's disease), Parkinson's disease, and Huntington's disease pose a particularly difficult challenge for caregivers. They're a clear exception to the notion that caregiving is not a burden. In part, the challenge stems from the fact that patients with advanced dementia and other neurologic conditions frequently need caregiving for years, even decades. Their diseases affect their thinking and can alter their personality and behavior. As dementia advances, patients may require close, full-time care so that they don't wander off or leave a pot boiling on the stove. Essentially, they can't be left alone. The cumulative burden of caring for those with advanced dementia and other neurologic conditions is depleting; it wears down caregivers. They endure what has been called the twenty-five-hour day.

Patients with advanced dementia may not treat their caregivers well. They can be maddeningly repetitive, inexplicably angry, intractable, demanding, unkind, and physically abusive. Out of the blue, quiet, elderly little women can curse like a sailor and strike out with astonishing venom and strength. People with advanced dementia frequently can't express their gratitude or remember past kindnesses. When they remain at home, their loved ones' health can be seriously jeopardized. Getting help with caregiving is especially important in this situation.

In some circumstances, caregiving becomes too much for family and friends, and patients may be better off in a facility. Making that decision can be agonizing, but it is often the best option all around.

As patients get sicker, they get weaker and find it harder to get around. Just moving them and getting them out of bed can take huge effort. Lifts and other equipment can help, and caregivers can learn strategies that make lifting easier and help them protect their bodies. Patients often end up in nursing homes or other care facilities because their loved ones are simply not strong enough to move them. As difficult as it can be, it is important to face our limitations.

Despite caregivers' best efforts, it can be difficult for them to be cheerful when they see their loved ones or clients decline. They may go through the five stages of grief that I discussed in chapter 1. As with patients, the stages for caregivers can be jumbled, come at different times, coexist, or overlap. Grief can affect caregivers' health, and they may need professional help during these difficult times.

It is important to recognize that illness takes a significant toll on caregivers that goes beyond the impact it has on them as family and friends. Professional caregivers also grieve; they're not immune to feeling profound sadness. In fact, the best caregivers care deeply about their patients and find it hard to watch them decline. It's an occupational hazard. Rest and taking care of themselves are essential to staying in the game.

WHEN HOME ISN'T THE PLACE

Some patients' needs are too great and/or their resources are not enough for them to remain at home. They may not have the space to accommodate the necessary equipment or simply can't make caregiving work at home. Still others may not want to be at home. The challenge is to find a place for them to live and get quality care. Nursing homes, assisted-living facilities, hospice residences, and board and care facilities are options. You also might be able to live in the home of another family member or a friend. When care at home won't work, your doctor or a social worker can help you find the best place to get the care you need.

Although patients in facilities such as hospitals, nursing homes, and hospices are cared for by many professionals, their family and friends can still help. As with Mrs. Chang, whose seven children took turns at her bedside while she was in the hospital, the presence of those who are familiar and trusted can be calming during a hospitalization or in a nursing home. Family and friends can also help you eat, get you drinks, and provide companionship. They can run errands and be another set of eyes and ears to observe what's going on, remember what the doctors and nurses say, and alert staff to changes or give them updates on how you're feeling. Family and friends can advocate for patients who may be too sick or reluctant to say that they're unhappy or uncomfortable. They can remind clinicians who the patient is as a person.

In the hospital, everything is different. People become patients: they're put in a gown and placed in an unfamiliar environment that they can't control. On top of all that, they're not at their best; they're sick. In the hospital, patients don't set the schedule, bathe regularly, sleep well, or eat what and when they normally would. They don't feel like themselves. Communication for the very sick, especially those on ventilators, may be difficult or impossible.

Clinicians often focus on the illness and can lose sight of the human, the unique individual, who is so ill: the father, grandmother, or aunt; the golfer, gardener, bus driver, or teacher in the bed. Who is he? What's she like? What does he do? Family and friends can give them background, share stories, and tell them who the patient is: his or her nature, character, and accomplishments.

Family and friends should bring in photos of their loved ones before they were hospitalized and show them to the staff. This will give them greater insight and understanding of the person in their care.

SUPPORT FOR CAREGIVERS

Caregiving is a risk factor for physical and psychological illness; when you provide care, you risk damaging your health. Caregivers also tend to ignore their own health issues, so they need to be sure they're paying attention to their well-being. Sleep, diet, and exercise are important and shouldn't be ignored. Since the patients they care for may be so much sicker than they are, they often see their problems as minor and expect them to go away. But their health issues may be more serious or become more serious if they're not addressed.

Support groups for caregivers and other types of help—hospice services, for example—can help caregivers. Data shows that spouses of patients who used hospice are less likely to die in the eighteen months after the patient dies [8.1]. Online caregiver support groups include Family Caregiver Alliance (www.caregiver.org), Caring.com (www.caring.com), Aging Care (www.agingcare.com), the AARP (www.aarp.org), Alzheimer's Association (www.alz.org), Smart Patients (www.smartpatients.com), and others.

CaringBridge (www.caringbridge.org) offers free, personalized websites for people who have serious medical conditions. They can set up a social-networking site for family members and friends to exchange information about the patient and to rally support for loved ones during a health journey.

Caregivers need support, so regardless of whether you're the patient or a family member, continually ask the caregivers, "How are you doing?" and "Can I help?" Showing your interest and letting them know that you care about them will help reduce their stress and help them feel better.

If you choose not to be hospitalized or to have every conceivable medical intervention, your choices may make some caregivers uncomfortable. If you and your caregiver have wildly different views on these issues, that person might not be the right caregiver for you. As I discuss in chapter 11, document your wishes and keep the documents in a prominent place in your home. Make sure that your caregiver is comfortable with your choices and committed to respecting them.

RX

Attitudes about caregiving are complicated. Some patients have strong feelings. They only want to be cared for by family members, and the thought of having a stranger in their home makes them very uncomfortable. They see hiring professional caregivers as a sign that their family and friends don't love them. Others can't imagine being cared for by family members; they think it's embarrassing and prefer professional caregivers.

Feelings also differ on giving care. Some see caregiving as a calling, an honor, and an expression of love and caring. They wouldn't dream of not providing care to their loved ones. Others find caregiving extremely stressful. They don't feel competent, worry about making mistakes, or just feel like they don't have it in them.

If you do become a caregiver, do your best and don't blame yourself or feel guilty about anything you did or didn't do. As with parenting, perfection is not required or possible, and good caregiving is great.

As in all aspects of life, and certainly in all issues involving serious illness, there is no one "right way." In order to live as well as possible with a serious condition, decisions about caregiving must be personalized. Find an approach that suits you and your family. If your family wants to care for you, do your best to let them. If they can't, do your best to understand and have compassion. As with most situations, talking it out and being clear about your preferences will lead to the best solution.

Finally, remember that caregiving is stressful, whether provided by family and friends or professionals. Take breaks, recharge, and make sure to take care of yourself. A burned-out caregiver means that two people need help. Know your limits, get more help, and remember that caregiving is a marathon, not a sprint.

chapter nine

THE NEWS GOES FROM BAD TO WORSE

SERIOUS ILLNESS IS A SERIES OF EVENTS, A PROCESS; IT'S not a single, isolated event. When you're seriously ill, it can seem like something new always occurs, and it's frequently not good. During your illness, you'll go through ups and downs, and your condition will change: at times it will be active, and at others it will be calm.

After the initial shock of your diagnosis and once you start treatment, you'll enter what I call a "new normal." Life will be different—sometimes very different—as you come to grips with your illness and what it means. In the new normal, uncertainty reigns; the unexpected occurs, and it becomes expected. After a while, you may feel as if you're fighting a string of fires: as soon as you put one out, another flares up.

Often, the news gets worse. It may happen suddenly and unexpectedly, and it may change everything. Let me give you some examples:

> › The CT scan taken after three months of chemotherapy shows that the cancer has spread, not shrunk.
> › After your heart attack, just as you're about to finish six weeks of cardiac rehabilitation, you land back in the hospital with shortness of breath and learn that your heart is weaker and your kidneys are failing.
> › You're at the top of the lung transplant list when you catch a cold. It puts you in the hospital and on a breathing machine, which disqualifies you for the transplant.

During serious illness, bad news piles up. It's like an El Niño—you have to weather a string of storms. At first, each deluge floors you and knocks you off your feet, but you get back up. Then it happens again, and again, and again. When you think that the news couldn't get worse, it does. Regardless of how prepared you are, how low your expectations may be, it's always a shock.

Bad news can also come out of the blue. You may be feeling great when things suddenly go bad. You're hit with new pain, more tumors, pneumonia, or blood clots. Each time you think, if I can just get through this, everything will be OK. As you treat those blood clots, however, you get pneumonia. As your pneumonia improves, you develop debilitating back pain. And as the back pain eases up, you fall and break a hip.

> At the same time, even during the fiercest storms, lulls occur. In the midst of the most violent battles, periods of calm exist. Savor the lulls; make the most of the interludes, the time between rounds. Use them to relax, reflect, reenergize, and regroup. Enjoy the days when you feel well, and don't overdo it.

When the complications pile up, the cumulative effect can be devastating and demoralizing. Individually, each complication may be fixable. Blood thinners treat blood clots, antibiotics work for pneumonia, physical therapy helps ease back pain, and hips can be fixed or replaced. Unfortunately, complications can add up and seem insurmountable.

DEALING WITH BAD NEWS

As the bad news piles up, acknowledge how rotten it feels. Think about it, live with it, let it sink in. Don't bury your disappointment, frustration, and fears. Then, when you've accepted your latest setback, plan to move forward.

I tell my patients that we have to take an honest look at the situation, see what cards we've been dealt, and decide the best way to play them. We can wish that we had a better hand, but we have to be realistic. We can't bluff. If we bet as if we have four aces when we have a pair of fives, we're going to lose big.

Playing the hand you've been dealt can be difficult because it means that you have to look at your cards clearly and realistically. You have to be honest and face the facts, which can take time to digest. It can be confusing, hard to grasp, and a reality that you don't want to accept. You had a plan—Plan A—but it didn't work out. The chemo didn't shrink your tumor; you aren't better, so you can't go back to work. So it's time to think about Plan B or Plan C.

Some patients think about alternative plans from the beginning. Some of my colleagues even suggest the idea to their patients early on. "Now that we have Plan A—you getting a liver transplant—let's think about a Plan B if you can't get the transplant in time." It can be hard to think about Plan B while you are counting on Plan A, and you may worry that thinking about

Plan B means that you're concerned that Plan A might not work. But considering alternative plans allows you to decide how you want to live and what you most want to accomplish, regardless of what happens.

Keep an eye on the big picture. When you see improvement in one area, it's tempting to tell yourself that everything is getting better, but that may not be realistic. In the ICU, we monitor every organ system and take lots of tests every day. Although some systems and some tests may be normal or even indicate some improvement, the overall picture can be poor and the patient may still be dying. I've heard colleagues tell the family of a dying patient, "Well, his kidneys are doing great." Talk about missing the forest for the trees.

> Even during setbacks, positives can also occur. Your condition could stabilize or improve. Even if you can no longer garden, you can sit in the garden and read a book. If you can't play your piano, you can listen to music on the radio or on CDs. You can also visit with family and friends, and watch your favorite movies. Appreciate what is going well—for example, that your pain is under control, your energy is back, or you're sleeping soundly. The mind excels at finding bright spots that can lift your spirits.

As hard as it can be, try to be realistic. Focus on whatever is stable or improving and appreciate it, but also accept what is not. If you feel emboldened, ask your doctor what it means that your kidneys are doing great when you're dying from cancer. Or perhaps you don't need to ask, because you already know that well-functioning kidneys can't cure your lung cancer but that the kidney specialist just can't find the right words to tell you that.

At some point, the bad news outweighs the good, and things get worse: you slow down, and you start spending more time in bed or in a chair. You go out less often. You stop gardening. You shorten your walks. Then you stop taking walks. You eat less and have less of an appetite. Little annoyances that you might have brushed off in the past, such as tripping on a stair or an ache in the back, suddenly become signs that something is seriously wrong. Although these changes tend to be gradual, they're distressing.

Most people take it hard. They get frustrated and scared. They sense that they're failing and want to fight. Unfortunately, these changes are caused by their illness, and they generally don't get better unless the underlying illness improves. When an illness gets worse, it's harder to reverse it or slow it down. When this happens, do the following:

> › Focus on what can make you feel better.
> › Make sure your pain is controlled.
> › If you have a poor appetite, identify foods you like and eat only those foods. Don't worry about low-fat this, low-carb that, or other restrictive diets. If all you want is ice cream, go for it. If you want to eat more, ask your doctor for medicines that can stimulate your appetite; just know that they won't make you stronger.
> › Do more of what you like and less of what you dislike.

Don't go through this process alone. Let others help you. Express your concerns to those who love you, who want what's best for you, and whose judgment you trust. Be honest and direct. Explain how you feel. Tell them your hopes and fears and solicit their advice. You may find strength and comfort in your spiritual or religious community.

> As difficult as this may be to read, it's important to be re-
> alistic, to know what you could be in for, so you can make
> the most of a raw deal. Yes, it will be difficult, but it will also
> open up opportunities for you. One such opportunity will be
> to ask yourself important questions, including assessing where
> you are, the path you're taking, and whether it's still helpful or
> if you want to change. Do you want to continue on the path
> you're following? If not, what are your options? What changes
> could make things better? Are they possible? What would mak-
> ing these changes involve?

Many of us are reluctant to bring up matters that are hard to
discuss or that may sadden others. It's human nature to avoid
these topics. You may worry that your loved ones won't respond
well, may shy away, or will say something inane, unhelpful, or
even hurtful. Although those responses are possible, those who
love you will be supportive; they'll usually respond better than
you had hoped. Discussing your feelings can bring you closer and
can ease your burden and theirs. I'm not suggesting that you have
these conversations with everyone or that you have them all the
time. Just talk to a few people who are closest to you, and not all
the time.

You may also be afraid to discuss changes that you've noticed in your body, as it could upset your loved ones. You may
also think that by not talking about the changes, they're not
happening, and as soon as you mention them out loud, you'll
make them real and undeniable. But talking about what is going
on can be a relief. It means you no longer have to try to cover
up or make excuses for the changes you notice. Talking does
not make it worse; in fact, getting it off your chest can make

you feel better. Your family will also feel better knowing that they can talk about what they noticed but were afraid to bring up with you.

When you talk about your condition, you can get information, allay fears, and take action. You may learn that the increased pain that you've felt recently isn't a sign that you're dying (it's not). Speak with your doctors. Ask tough, straightforward questions such as the following, and don't accept evasive answers.

> › "Where do I stand?"
> › "What does this mean for me?"
> › "What should I expect?"
> › "What would you suggest?"
> › "What can I do now?"
> › "How can I feel better?"

The answers you get may be jarring. They may be difficult to swallow, but learning the truth beats being in the dark. The truth will enable you to focus on reality and consider what may lie ahead. Then you can set your priorities and develop a plan to move forward.

Make decisions based on reality, not fantasy.

Marilyn, a sixty-two-year-old woman, had lung cancer that was no longer responding to chemotherapy and radiation. Each round had weakened her, and her cancer kept growing. Marilyn lived alone, had no family and only a few friends, and couldn't afford caregivers. She was in terrible pain that made her cry all the time, which she thought meant that she was dying. Marilyn worried about where she would live and who would take care of her. She was also eager to start a new cancer treatment that her oncologist recommended.

Our first order of business was pain control and assuring Marilyn that her pain didn't mean she was dying. When Marilyn was pain-free, we could focus on her cancer. A CT scan showed that the cancer had grown, which was not a surprise to Marilyn. We talked about what was most important to her. Marilyn's greatest concern was where she would live. She couldn't take care of herself anymore. We reviewed the options and discussed them. Together we agreed that a hospice unit would be the best place for her to get the care she needed.

On the morning she was to leave the hospital, Marilyn expressed doubts about whether to try the new cancer treatment. Could it extend her life? Make her stronger? Give her more energy? She was afraid that if she chose to get hospice care she would not be able to receive treatment for her cancer. When you have cancer, deciding to forgo chemo is hard. We realized that for Marilyn, as it is for most patients, it wasn't so much the chemo she was worried about, but admitting that she was approaching the end of life. Marilyn decided to move into a hospice residence. While there, she could visit her oncologist and discuss whether she should have the new cancer treatment. For the moment, she didn't need to choose.

Marilyn loved the hospice facility. She made fast friends with the staff and was calm and content. She forgot about the chemo. She played the hand she was dealt, and the path she took was the right one for her.

TREATMENT DECISIONS

When your illness advances, one of the most difficult decisions you face is whether to continue your present treatments or try new ones. Even if you opt not to continue treatments for your illness, you'll have to make other medical decisions because new treatments could become available to treat your illness and others could help manage complications such as blood clots and pneumonia.

Unfortunately, when your illness has advanced, you're usually not strong enough to get through difficult treatments. At that point, the chances that treatments will help you decrease because your illness has progressed and the risk of complications is greater. So be careful about agreeing to treatments while your condition deteriorates. Of course, it's when other options haven't succeeded that, in desperation, we consider throwing a Hail Mary pass.

I've seen patients respond well to experimental treatments, and I'm open to considering them, but go in with your eyes open and with a full understanding of the risks and benefits that could be involved (see chapter 3 for a discussion of Phase I clinical trials). More frequently, I've seen desperate people try treatments with the idea that "it couldn't get any worse," only to find that it indeed can get worse.

For example, if you undergo surgery, you'll have a surgical wound that will have to heal at a time when your body is weak and having difficulty healing. If you undergo general anesthesia, it will put your bowels to sleep and it will take time for them to wake up. You'll have to stay in the hospital for days or even weeks and run a higher risk of developing blood clots and serious infections. To make it worth it, the surgery has to have a good chance of making you substantially better.

It's hard to know with certainty whether you're in your last six months, so ask your doctor. And remember that doctors tend to be overly optimistic with prognosis. If you are at this point, think long and hard before agreeing to chemotherapy. If you have advanced heart disease, give careful consideration to more catheterizations or operations. And if your loved one has dementia and can

> A study of hundreds of cancer patients found that in the last six months of life, chemotherapy did not help them feel better or live longer. However, it did make a lot of them sicker. Those who were strongest at the outset saw their quality of life decline as a result of the chemotherapy [9.1].

no longer eat or drink, know that a feeding tube won't help him or her gain weight, get stronger, think better, or avoid pneumonia.

When you get bad news, it may not be the time to start new treatments. However, it may be the time to reconsider the treatments you're receiving. If, while you're undergoing treatments the news is bad, ask your doctor if you are getting the right treatments. Do you want to continue them?

While Ray was receiving monthly chemotherapy for colon cancer, he was also getting blood tests to monitor his carcinoembryonic antigen (CEA) level. At first, Ray's CEA went way down, which was good news; Ray's tumor was shrinking. But after several months, his CEA went up a bit.

Ray was worried. His doctor said not to panic and started Ray on different chemotherapy drugs. Ray, who wasn't the panicking kind, knew it didn't look good. Two months later, his CEA was up, but again it rose just a little. The doctor wasn't discouraged, but Ray saw the writing on the wall. His doctor managed to convince him to take one more dose, and despite Ray's better judgment, he agreed. A month later the CEA was way up. Ray was smiling when he told me, "I told the doctor three months ago that the chemo wasn't working. He just couldn't face it."

If you're committed to a treatment, it might be fine to continue it. Then again, it may not be. Each decision is unique and requires careful consideration. Ask yourself whether your regimen is helping you achieve your goal. Don't continue treatment out of habit or agree to treatments because you think you have no choice. You always have a choice, and the choice is yours alone.

Make practical decisions. For example:

> Don't return to the hospital if you hate it.
> Don't agree to surgery if it seems like it will be too much. Decline it or postpone your decision on it.
> Don't continue chemotherapy, radiation, or transfusions if they're wearing you down or simply because you've been undergoing them. Stop or take a break.

Mrs. Garner, a fifty-three-year-old woman, had advanced leukemia that made her extremely thin and weak. She ate little and spent most days in bed. Her bone marrow had been ravaged by chemotherapy, so she needed platelet transfusions three times a week to keep her from having life-threatening bleeding. The platelet transfusions had to take place in a medical center; we couldn't do them at home. Mrs. Garner's transfusions took up her entire day. She had to get ready, come to the medical center, get laboratory tests, wait for the platelets to be matched and prepared, get the transfusion, and return home. The whole process was exhausting, and Mrs. Garner needed the following day to recover. Then, the next day, she did it all over again. In all, she spent six days each week getting or recovering from transfusions and had only one day when she felt well.

Sadly, the transfusions didn't help Mrs. Garner. Her body destroyed the platelets almost as soon as they were infused, which is typical for people who have received multiple transfusions. Mrs. Garner was so tired that she couldn't enjoy time with her husband and children, which was the main reason she had agreed to the transfusions.

I saw Mrs. Garner when she was hospitalized for a new infection. I asked how she was holding up, and she said she was constantly tired. The trips to the hospital were wearing her out. I could tell that Mrs. Garner was not ready to stop the transfusions, so I suggested cutting back on the number she received each week, which would build her strength and give her more time at home.

At first, reducing the number of transfusions was hard for Mrs. Garner to even consider. She felt that fewer transfusions meant giving in, backing off her commitment to live. After a few days, Mrs. Garner decided to try two transfusions a week. The change worked: she felt better, gained more energy, and had more quality time to spend at home with her family.

Cutting back or declining treatments isn't giving up; it's not throwing in the towel. It doesn't mean that you're not battling or doing all you can to live. You have the right to choose the goals that have the greatest importance to you and to decide whether treatments will help you feel better. Sometimes, treatments meant to help make things worse.

Laura, a forty-two-year-old woman, had pancreatic cancer. She had undergone chemotherapy, but her cancer progressed. Laura had to drive nearly two hours for her treatments and to see her oncologist. Chemo made her sick and weak.

I saw Laura when she was admitted to the hospital with pain that we were able to quickly control. She told me that if it were up to her, she would never have chemo again. The way she said it struck me. I said, "It *is* up to you." She replied, "I guess, but it doesn't feel that way. My family is pushing me to try this new experimental treatment. They think if I don't then I'm giving up. I can't do it to them."

I wanted to cry for Laura. I hated to hear her tell me that if she didn't agree to have experimental chemotherapy, she would feel like she was letting her family down. It was especially hard to hear her say, "I can't do it to *them*" when she was the one who was taking all the risks, suffering, and facing death. Laura tried the chemotherapy. It made her very sick, and she stopped after one dose.

The decision about whether to undergo experimental chemotherapy was a great—but lost—opportunity for Laura and her family to talk. They could have discussed Laura's situation as well as her and her family's concerns. By talking, they could have forged understanding, strengthened bonds, and built indelible memories, which would have been a great gift. They could have shown unity, felt togetherness, and made it clear that they shared the same hopes, objectives, and concerns. If they had spoken with Laura, her family could have demonstrated their love and support and heard her concerns.

Family and friends must recognize when to push and when to hold back. They are motivated by love; they have the best intentions. They hope that encouraging their loved ones to have more treatments and to try new and experimental thereapies will help them feel better and live longer. However, they frequently don't realize how much pressure they put on those who are already suffering.

As a friend or family member, say, "I love you and want what's best for you. It's hard for me to think of not trying everything to treat your illness, but I support you and what is most important to you. What can I do to help you?"

I've cared for many patients from cultures where decisions about treatment are not individual but family based. The primary concern is what would be best for the family, not for the patient. I respect that point of view. Yet, even in those situations, patients and their families still have room to talk, to discuss their wishes and goals. The fact that a treatment decision was made by your family doesn't mean it has to be for more interventions and more treatment. It also doesn't mean that your family will continue to make all treatment decisions and that you, the patient, will have no input. Speak up. It's your illness, your life. Talk with them, because the benefits of talking far outweigh the awkwardness and discomfort it might cause.

Stopping treatments can be hard because it may mean that you no longer go to the clinic or hospital, which was a source of support and connection. You may feel a sense of loss when you no longer see your doctors, nurses, and medical team. Treatments can also give you a purpose and structure, a reason to get out of bed and get dressed. Taking treatments is also a sign that you're being proactive, taking action to deal with your illness, even though the odds of their helping may be slim.

On the other hand, discontinuing treatment has benefits. You may gain energy that you previously expended going to hospitals, infusion centers, or clinics. You also get more time and freedom from lines, tubes, needle jabs, and the side effects of treatments.

When you stop going to places where sick people congregate, your risk of complications shrinks because medical facilities house lots of nasty bacteria. Although we constantly scour them with powerful disinfectants, dangerous bugs remain and patients continually bring in more. Staying away from hospitals, clinics, and infusion and dialysis centers lowers your chances of catching something dangerous and potentially deadly. You can still stay connected to your doctor and nurses. You can visit your doctor even if you are not continuing treatments. You can also talk by phone and possibly even arrange for a home visit.

In the study of palliative care for lung cancer patients conducted by my friend and colleague Dr. Jennifer Temel [9.2], the researchers concluded that one reason patients who received palliative care lived longer might be because they avoided treatments like chemotherapy and hospitalizations that might have caused complications and made them sicker.

NEW AND INCREASING PAIN

Patients with serious illness worry that they will be in pain, and with good reason. Pain is awful and common for people with serious illness, though not universal. We all know that pain is a signal that something's wrong and that we should address it. So it frightens us, makes us tense and upset, which can increase our suffering and impede healing.

During serious illness, patients can get new pains and their existing pain can increase. It's inherent when most illnesses progress, though not inevitable. Patients often take it as a sign that they're nearing the end. However, that's not necessarily so. As I pointed out in chapter 6, pain is not a prognostic sign, and new or more-intense pain does not mean you're about to die—even from cancer.

The fact that your new or increasing pain isn't fatal doesn't mean that you shouldn't address it. Addressing it is imperative. Contact your doctors promptly because they can treat your pain and frequently provide relief. Treatment helps you function better all around. Although addressing your pain won't cure your illness or restore you to your former good health, it may give you more strength, energy, and motivation to get through your illness and optimize your time.

You can't get help unless you ask for it. So when you get new pains or your existing pains increase, ask your medical team for help. Don't be one of those people who won't ask for help because they think that they'll be admitting that their condition is deteriorating. Yes, new and worsening pain frequently signifies that you're sicker, but not always. Speak with your doctor and get the facts. Don't be a martyr and don't live in denial. Get help. Suffering is pointless and unnecessary.

RX

I've previously emphasized that I don't believe that serious illness is a gift. Serious illness is dreadful, and going through it is painful and sad. Declining health can be even worse. Good health is always better. Most people say that they would like to die in their sleep at a very old age without ever being sick. I'd like the same for myself. But for most of us, life won't work that way. It's more likely that we'll live with a serious illness that may last for months, years, or even decades. That's the norm. Given that fact, it is worth asking what good can come from your illness—to concentrate on the good, the positive, rather than the bad.

This perspective is the gift I often refer to. Ask yourself, "Today, in my current situation, what good could come my way? What changes could I make? What unfinished business could I finish, what broken friendships could I repair, or what wrongs could I right?"

Savor the little things, embrace special moments, and appreciate your blessings. Be open, forgive, explore, and change. Spend your time freely and generously on yourself, on those you love, on those in need, and on doing what you care about most.

Every morning, Marilyn would say how grateful she was to no longer be in pain and to feel secure. Her gratitude didn't change the fact that she was dying; nothing could change that. But it did give her moments of respite and calm. Gratitude helps us feel better. You can't feel angry and grateful at the same time. Focus on gratitude by asking yourself, "What am I grateful for today?"

I recommend that every day, my patients and their loved ones write three things that they're grateful for that day. It always helps me.

chapter ten

BIG CONCEPTS, WORDS, AND GOALS

YOUR VALUES AND BELIEFS SHAPE WHO YOU ARE. THEY affect how you live, how you get through your illness, and the legacy you leave. When you're healthy and engaged in your busy life, details and deadlines tend to dominate your time. You think that your time frame is long, that you can plan well into the future and can engage in activities that may take years, even decades, to bear fruit. Day after day, you take care of business; one by one, you cross items off your list only to see new ones quickly take their place.

As you attend to each day's needs, you slip into a zone. You zero in on each pressing problem and emergency; you get lost in them. You're on a mission to complete each task excellently and efficiently, so you attack them fully, whole-heartedly. As you do, things you hold most dear can be pushed aside; they can fall victim to expediency and slip through the cracks.

When you're seriously ill, your perspective changes. Your focus shifts. Matters that you treated lightly or took for granted become more important to you, and concerns that barely interested you now top your list. What you value most takes on greater meaning.

Serious illness also forces you to make difficult and important decisions. When those decisions are matters of life and death, your deeply held values and beliefs guide you. They rush to the surface and clarify what's most important to you.

When your mind is clear, making decisions isn't a big deal. It's what we do every day. However, during serious illness, it's harder to make informed decisions regarding your treatment and your future for a number of reasons.

First, you may not have enough information. The information you need may be too technical or simply unknown; all the possible outcomes may not be clear. You may be offered a treatment that hasn't been tested on others in your situation, or you may be asked to choose between two paths that both have major risks. Treatments that can have terrible side effects could be your only hope. You may feel like you have no good options.

As Roger's stomach cancer grew, it started to bleed. Occasionally, it bled a lot and Roger had to come to the hospital for transfusions and close monitoring. Then Roger developed blood clots in his leg and lung that were life threatening. The treatment for blood clots is taking blood thinners, which would increase Roger's risk of bleeding. Roger agonized over whether to take blood thinners, and after evaluating the alternatives, he finally decided to take them because his risk of dying from the clot was greater than his risk of bleeding to death. We gave Roger a blood thinner that would be quick and easy to reverse, and although he had more bleeding, it fortunately wasn't too severe.

Second, you may not have much time to think about your decisions. Many medical decisions have to be made quickly. For example, blood thinners for an embolism must be given as soon as possible, or the clots could break off and cause harm or even death. Other decisions, including those about intubation, may have to be made in minutes. Some decisions, however, can be made in advance, which I'll discuss in chapter 11.

Third, you may be too sick, too weak, or too tired to make important treatment decisions. Others may have to make them on your behalf, which I'll also cover in chapter 11. Since it's impossible to know if and when these situations will occur, act beforehand if possible: anticipate the worst and decide how you want to proceed. Then tell your doctors and your loved ones what you want.

Making major decisions about our health and treatment is difficult. Even just thinking about it is hard. It's something none of us want to do—until we must. Most of us are unprepared and don't know where to start. We're on new ground, foreign territory, a place we've never been.

Get the best information you can and trust your gut. Some people avoid risk; they don't want to make decisions that could turn out to be harmful. Others are risk takers. They'll try anything and everything that they think might help. When complications arise, some people will be comfortable knowing that they took action, and others will blame themselves. In these situations, no right or wrong answer exists. If the evidence was clear, your doctor would have told you. You can ask for recommendations, but your decisions must be based on what is most important to you—after all, you're the one undergoing treatment. Good decisions require frank conversations with your medical team.

After you make a decision, don't second-guess or blame yourself. If complications arise, try to find the best way to move forward. In my family, we talk about "NBA": the next best action.

THE BIG PICTURE

To make the best decisions, focus on the big picture and identify the goals you would like to reach; prioritize what you would like to accomplish most. By goals I mean big picture objectives and end results, not the individual tasks that get you there.

Patients tell me that their goal is to get radiation, get an implant, or undergo certain procedures, but I don't consider those to be goals. They're means toward achieving goals. Goals are spending more time with family, completing your book, visiting your hometown, selling your business, completing graduate school, getting your child settled at college, and making amends with your sister. Medical interventions are means for achieving your goals.

As I discussed in chapter 3, it's important to know whether your goal is achievable. Push your doctors to tell you. I've cared for many patients who agreed to undergo aggressive and difficult treatments in the hope that they would be cured. Had they inquired and known from the outset that a cure was not possible, they may have decided not to take those treatments.

Treatments that you hope will help you achieve your goals may backfire on you. They may undermine your goals and prevent you from reaching what you want most. Too often, I've seen patients go through courses of grueling chemotherapy in order to live better and longer and have more time with their children, only to get sicker from the chemotherapy and have less time with those they love. Their chemo made their immune systems so weak that they couldn't be around their children, who could expose them to minor colds—colds that could be deadly for them. They ended up in the hospital, too weak to hold their babies and too sick to be with their children. Treatments that were supposed to give them more time with their families actually did the opposite.

Similarly, families often request feeding tubes for patients with advanced dementia who are not eating. They think that forced feeding will help their loved one live longer, gain weight, get stronger, or avoid pneumonia. However, feeding tubes don't achieve any of those objectives in patients with advanced dementia. Careful feeding by hand works better. Not eating occurs naturally with advanced dementia patients; it is a sign that their bodies are shutting down, not the cause of their bodies' failure.

Think about your goals. Talk with family and friends. I ask my patients, and encourage you to ask yourself, the following:

> "What is most important to me right now?"
> "What is left undone?"

Speak with your doctor. Discuss which treatments will help you achieve your goals. Then make a plan to reach them.

> *"A goal without a plan is a wish."*
> —Antoine de Saint-Exupéry

While setting clear goals is crucial, be careful not to set unattainable ones. It's natural to want to shoot for the stars when the stakes are so high. But it's also important to recognize when pursuing impossible goals will simply distract you from living well today and rob you of achieving other important goals that are attainable. When you're seriously ill, it's important not to joust at windmills.

Pursuing unrealistic goals can set you back. It wastes time, energy, and valuable resources—resources that are in short supply and not renewable. Once they're spent, they're gone. Hopes and dreams act as incentives and give you purpose, but when they have no chance of being realized, they squander your resources. Chasing promises of being cured from clinic to clinic and undergoing risky treatments that won't help you achieve your goal can break your spirit, your health, your heart, and your bankroll. It can also devastate those who love you.

If you have multiple goals, reaching all your goals may be impossible, so prioritize. Decide what you want most. Your goals might be to stay at home, have your pain controlled, and be awake and clear enough to spend meaningful time with family and friends. It may be possible to achieve all three goals simultaneously, but often it's not. When push comes to shove, your priorities may be to: (1) have your pain well controlled, (2) be awake and clear and have meaningful time with family and friends, and (3) stay at home. You may reach a point when having your pain well controlled might mean you are not awake or that you can't stay at home. On the other hand, if staying at home and being awake were more important to you, you might be willing to accept slightly less pain control. A big part of what our palliative care team does is come up with creative solutions to help people achieve as many of their goals simultaneously as possible.

Prognosis plays an important role in goal setting. The goals you can reasonably achieve will depend on your prognosis, as will how you prioritize those goals. They'll change, depending on whether you have a few months, a year, or five years to live.

Your goals don't have to be set in stone. They can, and probably will, change as your condition and circumstances change. That is to be expected. Keep the conversation going.

BIG CONCEPTS

Big concepts form and give shape to the big picture. They help you identify, develop, and define your goals. Talking about concepts and goals, discussing them with others, helps you refine them. It clarifies them in your mind, which impacts your decision making and makes it easier. Discussing how you think about these important concepts and goals helps others understand and remember what's important to you.

When you talk about big concepts, it's important that you clarify what you mean. People have different ways of defining the same concept. Think about the concepts listed below and define what each means to you.

Dignity: Let's start with the concept of dignity. Dignity is one of the most common and passionately advocated concepts that I hear from patients, their loved ones, and doctors. They believe that it's essential to preserve the dignity of those who are seriously ill. I completely agree. However, it's not clear precisely what they mean because dignity has different meanings to different people, and wildly different decisions can be made in the pursuit of dignity.

Dignity is defined as "inherent nobility; self-respect that inspires honor and esteem." Every human being has innate dignity, and serious illness can feel like an affront to it. Many patients tell me that if their illnesses will make them dependent on others (for example, in need of help with bodily functions) or limit their cognitive abilities, they will feel a loss of dignity. On the other hand, other patients feel that these issues have no connection to their sense of dignity. For them, their dignity is inherent in who they are and is not related to what they are able or not able to do physically. It is no surprise that nearly all the seriously ill patients I treat tell me how important dignity is to them. They all want to maintain their dignity.

But what does dignity mean in the context of serious illness? For some it means that life is sacred, and they should maintain life for as long as possible—even if it takes the assistance of machines and even if they can no longer speak or interact. For others, being connected to machines in the ICU and unable to engage with the world would be a complete loss of dignity.

Just before she died, my mother told our family, "Please stay with me as I die. But after I die and before they come to take my body, leave the room. I don't want you to be there when they remove my body." She wanted us to be with her until she died but not to see her lifeless body, which offended her sense of dignity.

Dignity therapy: My friend Dr. Harvey Max Chochinov, the author of *Dignity Therapy* (Oxford University Press, 2012), has conducted research on dignity at the end of life and has developed dignity therapy to support and promote dignity for seriously ill patients. In dignity therapy, a patient with serious illness is asked what she values, what she thinks is most important, and what she wants her loved ones to remember. Her answers are recorded, transcribed, and edited to make them easy to read. The document is printed and reviewed with the patient. When the patient approves it, as they almost always do, they are given a copy of a finalized document to share with their loved ones.

Harvey's research found that discussing dignity makes patients feel better. It provides an increased sense of purpose and meaning. Below are some of the questions asked. Consider these questions and share your answers with your loved ones.

> When did you feel most alive?
> What are the most important roles you have played in your life and why are they so important to you?
> What are your most important accomplishments and of what do you feel most proud?
> What are your hopes and dreams for your loved ones?
> What advice or words of guidance would you wish to pass along?

As I pointed out in chapter 4, doctors can also be unclear when they use the word *dignity*. They often refer to dignity when recommending that invasive treatments be stopped, especially for patients in the ICU. They assume that invasive treatments violate patients' dignity and that stopping them and letting the patients die would restore and honor the patients' dignity. Not all families see it that way. Dignity is a concept we need to talk about in order to fully understand its meaning to different people.

Quality of life: What does "having the best quality of life" mean to you? We all want to have a good quality of life, and the goal of medicine is to help people have the best quality of life possible.

However, we're not great judges of what gives quality to other people's lives. We don't know how they define "quality of life" or what it means to them.

To a twenty-year-old, quality of life may mean being able to ski double black diamond runs. But finding an eighty-year-old who defines it that way is rare. A study that investigated quality of life compared the feelings of lottery winners and people who were paralyzed [10.1]. As you might expect, those who were paralyzed were not quite as happy as the lottery winners, but the difference was small. People in both groups found about the same amount of happiness from everyday experiences like talking with friends, and they thought that they would be happy in the future in equal measure. We humans have a remarkable capacity to find quality in our lives.

We know from other studies that sick people tend to value their quality of life more than their loved ones or doctors and nurses. The meaning of quality of life is subjective. Each of us must determine what it means to us. No one else can define it for us. So don't leave it up to others to decide what a good quality of life would be for you. Tell your loved ones. Give them examples of the quality of life you would like.

A patient once told me that as long as he could watch football on TV and enjoy it, he'd consider that an acceptable quality of life. More commonly, patients will say that being unable to recognize family members and interact meaningfully would be a quality of life that they wouldn't want to continue. Another patient told me, "When I can't tell you directly that my quality of life is good, then it's not."

Ask yourself:

> What does quality of life mean to me?
> What gives my life quality?

› What is most important to have in my life in order to give
   it quality?

› What would make me think that I no longer have a good
   enough quality of life?

Write down your answers. Think about them when you're
making treatment decisions. Then discuss them with loved ones
so they will have clear guidance on decisions they may have to
make on your behalf. I'll address this more in chapter 11.

Legacy: Think about what you will leave to others and the world
as a result of your having been alive. How do you hope to be
thought of and remembered? What will you be grateful for, regret, want to resolve or have closure on?

As you approach the end of life, you may find it rewarding to
review what you've accomplished, your exploits, and what you
consider important. Sharing your experiences and feelings with
your family can be enjoyable and affirming. The stories of your
life from childhood to the present, what you've been through,
could fascinate others, open their eyes, and give them insights
and guidance. These stories can shape how you will be remembered and live on.

For many, their children are their greatest legacy. For others,
it's work, teaching, mentoring, protecting, volunteering, or being a
good and loyal friend. For most of us, our legacy will be our acts of
kindness and how we touched and helped others, our community,
and the world. Few of us will leave a legacy of great literature, art,
or political success; we won't be remembered as Olympic athletes
or movie stars. How we lived our lives and our personal and intimate relationships will be the gifts we leave behind.

Part of your legacy will be the lessons you've learned that you
can pass on to others: your values, your beliefs, what you hold

dear, and what you stand for. Clarify your legacy by considering these questions:

> What are the secrets of a good life?
> What does it mean to be a good person?
> What have you done that you're proud of?
> What is the meaning of life?
> If you could live your life over, what would you do differently?

When you reflect on your legacy, you'll confront the ways in which you may have failed to live up to your values and not fulfilled your dreams. Forgive yourself. The lessons you learned and the reasons you fell short could rectify your failure and prove valuable to your loved ones. It may give you the opportunity to make amends and set things right.

At a time in your life when illness may prevent you from doing so much of what gave your life meaning and joy—working, traveling, volunteering, and caring for others—sharing your values, the discoveries you made, the processes you went through, and the secrets of your success can be a way that you contribute to the world. For many, speaking openly and sincerely about these topics provides tremendous gratification and meaning.

WHAT IS MOST IMPORTANT?

Here's a story I love. It's about understanding and identifying what's most important.

A professor stood before her philosophy class and picked up a large, empty glass jar. She filled the jar with stones. Then the professor asked her students if the jar was full. They all said yes. So she took a box of pebbles and poured them into the jar. She shook the jar lightly, and the pebbles settled into the spaces between the stones. When she asked her students if the jar was now full, they all enthusiastically said yes.

Then the professor poured fine sand into the jar, and it slipped into the gaps between the pebbles and the stones. Before she could ask, her students yelled that yes, the jar was full. The professor then took two cups of coffee and poured them into the jar. As the coffee filled the jar and dripped over the top, the students laughed.

"This jar represents your life," the professor said. "The stones are what is most important—your family, your health, your friends, and your passions. If everything else was lost and only they remained, your life would still be full. The pebbles are other things that matter, like your house, your possessions, and your hobbies. The sand is all the small stuff."

"If you put the sand into the jar first, you'll have no room for the stones or the pebbles. The same is true in your life. If you spend all your effort on the small stuff, you'll never have room for what is really important. Focus on the things that are of the greatest importance to you. Spend time with friends and family. Take care of your body. Do whatever you're most passionate about. You can always find time to clean the house, answer emails, and take out the trash. Focus on the stones, the things that really matter. The rest is just sand."

A student raised her hand and asked about the coffee. The professor smiled. "I'm really glad you asked. It just goes to show that no matter how full your life may seem, there's always room for a cup of coffee with a friend."

> What are the stones in your life?
> Are you making time for coffee?
> Stop worrying about the sand.

Serious illness, especially as it advances, is difficult. It's a time of slowing down, when our bodies fail and fall apart. As you go through your illness, it can seem as if nothing good lies ahead and that you're just waiting for the next setback to occur. Although many losses come with serious illness, it can also be a time of personal growth and development. It can help you focus on what you've accomplished and what you want to leave behind.

ETHICAL WILLS

Documents that capture your story, your values, and/ or the lessons you've learned are called ethical wills. They don't convey your material possessions but express your values and beliefs. They also may contain your hopes for the future and messages of love and forgiveness. A long history of ethical wills exists in many cultures, stretching back to ancient Hebrew and Christian traditions. According to the Hebrew Bible, Jacob gathered his children at his deathbed to express his thoughts on how best to live.

Just as children must take on developmental tasks, seriously ill people have to consider and complete certain tasks. As I've said, an important task is to share the story of your life. Another task is to bring closure to significant relationships. One of our greatest fears about dying is not having the opportunity to bring closure to relationships.

Serious illness is a time to think about your relationships and how you want to attend to them. In his book *Dying Well* (Riverhead Books, 1997), my friend Dr. Ira Byock offers five statements we should say to those we care about to bring closure:

Forgive me.
I forgive you.

Thank you.

I love you.

Good-bye.

Often, we don't know what to say to those who are ill. My patients tell me that they don't know exactly what to say to their loved ones either. These five statements say it all. They're short, simple, and heartfelt. They express regret, forgiveness, gratitude, and love and provide closure by saying good-bye.

When I outlined these statements with the son of one of my dying patients, he looked at me and ticked off each one. "Done that," he said. "And that, that, and that. I guess it's time to say good-bye."

RX

Serious illness is a series of decisions. Those decisions are not primarily about treatments; they're about what is most important to you. What you believe to be most important comes from your values and goals. Focus on the stones, not the sand. It will help you make decisions that you'll be comfortable with and that will feel right to you. As you get sicker, your values and goals will become even more important guideposts. They can help you find greater comfort and peace.

Concentrate on the big picture. Get the information you need and ask the tough questions. You'll have many goals. Some of them will conflict. Prioritize and realize that your goals will change over time. Solidify your thinking by defining what quality of life means to you.

PART III

looking ahead

chapter eleven

THE GIFT: PLANNING YOUR FUTURE SO YOUR LOVED ONES DON'T HAVE TO

WE KNOW THAT OUR DEATH IS INEVITABLE, THAT SOONER or later we may be hit with a serious illness that could turn our lives upside down. Although we know it's coming, most of us do nothing; we don't even bring up the subject to those who are the closest and most important people in our lives. Ignoring this reality is a cultural phenomenon.

In a survey released in 2012 [11.1], the California Health Care Foundation (CHCF) found that 60 percent of adults surveyed said that "making sure my family is not burdened by tough decisions about my care" was "extremely important," but 56 percent had not communicated their wishes. The survey, titled "Final Chapter: Californians' Attitudes and Experiences with Death and Dying," also found that 82 percent of those surveyed said that if they were seriously ill, it would be important for them to put their wishes in writing, but only 23 percent had done so. More than half said that they had not talked with a loved one about the kind of care they would want at the end of life.

Nearly eight out of ten respondents said that they would want to speak with their doctor about end-of-life care, but just 7 percent had had that conversation, including just 13 percent of those who were sixty-five or older. According to those surveyed, one of the most important factors at the end of life was "making sure that my family is not burdened financially by the costs of my care." This concern was followed closely by "being comfortable and without pain."

Although the disparity between what people want and what they actually do is striking, the survey also revealed another distressing problem: most patients' preferences are not followed. Only 44 percent of those who lost a loved one in the last twelve months said that the deceased's preferences were completely followed and honored by medical providers. When language barriers existed, the rate fell to only 26 percent. In addition, of the 70 percent who said that they wanted to die at home, only 32 percent actually did.

Sadly, the CHCF survey shows that odds are that your wishes will not be honored. You will probably get care you don't want and from which you won't benefit, such as chemotherapy in the last months of your life, and fail to receive care you do want from which you would benefit, like excellent pain control. If you're seriously ill, the best way to improve your odds is by thinking about your wishes in advance and telling your loved ones what you want. Find the time to let them know what's most important to you. Explain how you would like to live, be treated, and die, and even what you want done with your body after you die. Although these conversations are difficult and awkward, they're necessary. Without them, the care you receive probably won't be the care you want.

AN ACT OF LOVE

Giving clear directions is a gift, an act of love. Your loved ones may have to make agonizing decisions at the worst, most highly charged emotional times. Not expressing your wishes will leave them guessing, and they could guess wrong. Without guidance, your loved ones will have to figure out what you wanted and could end up making important decisions on the basis of their emotions, beliefs, wants, and/or needs, which may differ from yours. What is even harder on your loved ones is that lack of direction from you can burden your survivors, leave them feeling guilty, and increase the emotional and practical impact of your loss.

Directives can make your wishes clear. They let everyone know what you value and want. Clear directives help to avoid potential problems that could divide your loved ones. Without clear directives, the loudest, most forceful, or most conservative voices may seize control, and those who have to make decisions may feel overwhelmed, agonize over decisions, and feel guilty about them. Remaining silent can create confusion and cause family disputes that can be gut wrenching, costly, and divisive.

Doctors are trained to keep patients alive, and emergency rooms and hospitals do everything to keep you going—unless you make it clear that you want something different. Without clear directions that state your preferences, you could be subjected to unnecessary pain, discomfort, and financial costs. Advance health care directives and a forceful advocate to speak on your behalf are the best ways to make sure that your wishes will be respected.

KEY DECISIONS

Planning for your future accomplishes two objectives. First, you give your loved ones guidance on how to make medical decisions for you if you reach a point where you're unable to make those decisions for yourself. Second, you anticipate possible scenarios and reflect on your values and goals so that when the time comes to make medical decisions, which could be tomorrow or in months or years, you're clear about what is most important to you.

Sometimes doctors approach these as two separate processes, though they tend to blur and overlap. We call the first process advance care planning—planning for the future when you may be too sick to speak on your own behalf. This process is meant to guide your loved ones and doctors should you end up in a dire medical situation and be too sick to speak.

The second process is called goals of care. It aims to clarify your goals and identify care and treatments that will help you achieve those goals. When you're healthy, it's really all about advance care planning. If you were in a car accident or suffered a massive stroke and were not conscious, your loved ones would have instructions on the type of care you want and the values that should guide your care. As you get sicker, decisions about treatments become more immediate; they're no longer far off in the future. Goals of care focus on your goals, and those goals guide treatments. Of course, the decisions you make today will also guide your care in the future.

Another essential decision in planning your future is choosing who will speak for you if you become unable to speak for yourself. This person is known as your surrogate. Choose your surrogate carefully because whom you choose could be the most important decision you make.

STEP 1: CHOOSE YOUR SURROGATE

The three criteria for a good surrogate are as follows:

1. Trusting your surrogate to carry out your wishes.
2. Choosing a person who knows you well and whom you have spoken to about your preferences and goals.
3. Knowing that he or she will be available when needed.

First and foremost, select a surrogate who you can rely on to carry out your wishes. Many people can't make these difficult decisions, and they shouldn't be forced to. Make sure the person you choose is willing to serve. I've had people tell me that they need their daughter to be their surrogate because they know their son won't be able to make the tough decisions to decline invasive interventions. It can be hard to choose one person over another. Does that mean you love someone more? No, but it can feel that way to the person not chosen. These conversations are difficult. Not just because of the issues you have to talk about but because you may be choosing between people you love. But the stakes are high, and you want to get it right.

Some people choose a committee—"My five children will make a decision together"—or simply don't choose a surrogate. If you don't choose a surrogate, the doctors and nurses will look to your family to help make medical decisions if you are too sick to speak for yourself. In many states, a law designates who has priority to serve as your surrogate if you don't choose one in advance.

Be careful about leaving decisions to a committee or to the legally designated individual. What tends to happen is that your loved ones try to reach consensus, and if one person is not comfortable or is louder or more forceful, the rest defer. Very often, keeping peace in the family trumps the patient's wishes, or your loved ones simply can't agree on what you would want and the decision defaults to you receiving more interventions. This is another way that people end up with care they don't want at the end of life. You probably already know who could make the tough decisions. Choose that person. And let everyone else know whom you have chosen so there is no confusion later.

> A rule regarding surrogates: Anyone can be your surrogate, with a few exceptions. Your doctor can't be your surrogate and neither can anyone who works for your doctor or the hospital or nursing home where you get care, unless that person is related to you by blood or marriage.

STEP 2: TALK ABOUT YOUR GOALS, VALUES, AND PREFERENCES WITH YOUR SURROGATE

To be an effective spokesperson representing your wishes, which is what a surrogate is supposed to do, your surrogate needs to know you well, and you need to talk with him or her about your preferences, goals, and feelings about quality of life. If you just can't pick one person, talk with your "committee" about your preferences and goals. Unless you discuss these matters directly, your surrogate may end up guessing and could guess wrong. Even close family and friends find it difficult to know what your goals and preferences are without an explicit conversation.

As I discussed in chapter 10, think about your goals. Ask yourself:

> What is most important in my life?
> What do I hope will happen?
> What is worrying me the most?

Tell your surrogate, as specifically as possible, what you would like. Describe the quality of life you prefer and would accept, and express your feelings about hospitalization. Specify the treatments you don't want. For example, say whether you want a feeding tube, CPR, mechanical ventilation, and antibiotics and under what conditions.

You can't anticipate everything that might happen. During serious illness, surprises constantly occur, and everything doesn't always go as planned. That's why it's so important for your surrogate to understand your values and beliefs and to have the strength to implement them. Then, if everything goes haywire or they have to make decisions on matters that you didn't cover, they'll know what to do. They'll come to the same conclusions you would have and make decisions consistent with your values.

STEP 3: MAKE SURE YOUR SURROGATE IS AVAILABLE

Surrogates don't necessarily have to be present in person, but they must be able and willing to pick up the phone any time, day or night, to speak with your doctors. This is a serious responsibility and should not be taken lightly. Since your surrogate may not always be available, also appoint an alternate to serve when your surrogate cannot. Discuss your preferences and goals with your alternate as well.

IF YOU'RE THE SURROGATE

If you're a surrogate for a loved one and are asked to help doctors make a medical decision, ask yourself, "What would your loved one say if he or she were listening in on the call or sitting next to me?" I often prompt surrogates by asking a question such as, "If your mom were here with us and could tell us what she thinks of what is happening to her right now, what would she say?" The best answer always starts, "My mom and I talked about this, and if she were here she would say . . . " or "My mom and I didn't discuss this exact situation, but we did talk about what was most important to her, and based on that discussion she would want. . . ."

With all the stress and emotions involved in helping to make medical decisions as a surrogate, it can be easy to get a bit confused as to what you should do. Sometimes I'll start with the basics and ask, "Tell me about your mom. What was she like? What was important to her?" The answers often clarify what their loved one would have said.

Surrogates may put themselves in their loved one's situation. Surrogates and family members will often say, "If it were me, this is what I would do" or "I would never want to live like that." I try to acknowledge the importance of their responses and provide some context: "Thank you for sharing that. It is very interesting to know how you would decide for yourself, but that's not what we're here to talk about. We're here to talk about what your mom would say about this situation."

When I'm discussing a particular treatment or procedure, I try to help surrogates by asking them if the patient ever talked to them about that procedure—for example, a feeding tube. Often they have. They read about it, saw something on the TV or Internet, or know someone who went through it and talked about it. Such information can be very helpful. As a surrogate, ask yourself the same questions while you're trying to decide what your loved one would have wanted.

As a surrogate, be prepared for "the call." Frequently, it comes in the middle of the night from someone you've never met and requires an immediate answer. Does your loved one want to be intubated or receive ICU-level care? What are his or her goals?

Take a moment. Sit down. Catch your breath. Someone may ask you, "What do you want us to do?" Ask what the choices are, what the various outcomes would be, and how likely each is. It may be hard to think, but do your best to ask questions so you can understand what is going on. If you have even a few minutes and your loved one has a doctor who knows him or her and whom you trust, call that doctor.

BE CLEAR ABOUT YOUR GOALS

Clarity is crucial. The clearer you can be about your goals, the more likely they will be honored and respected. When you give directions, be as clear and precise as possible. State exactly what you mean. Give examples and instructions and emphasize what you want.

"I don't want to be a vegetable": Patients tell me that they would accept ICU care and intubation, but they don't want to be a "vegetable." The trouble is, the word *vegetable*, when applied to someone who is sick, isn't precise, and frankly, it's seldom a word we use in medicine (there is a diagnosis called a "persistent vegetative state," and it is rare and has very specific criteria). I worry that patients think we know exactly what they mean. When I hear that term, I ask my patients to explain. "What does it mean to you to be a vegetable?" "What would be the worst part of it?"

I wouldn't want my children to choose the music I listen to or the clothes I wear without my guidance. Sure, they know me; they know what I listen to and my style of dressing. But I wouldn't leave those choices to them. Some of their ideas about the kind of music I should listen to or the kind of clothes I should wear could creep in. The same goes for medical care, which is a thousand times more important. If my children get a song or shirt wrong, that's of little consequence. However, if they get my preferences for medical care wrong, I could be in for a long and painful ride that I never wanted. And the burden of making medical decisions could weigh heavily on them. I love my boys and don't want them to struggle with making decisions about my care without my guidance. I don't want them to worry about getting it wrong or feeling guilty. Turns out I'm pretty good at telling them how I think things should go. No reason to stop when it comes to my care.

Lack of clear, explicit direction can be agonizing and can force decision makers to go through unnecessary discomfort. When decision makers have little or no guidance, they can worry about whether they made the best decisions. Doubts can linger for years. Lack of direction can also lead to their erring on the side of doing more than you wanted.

You can't anticipate everything that might happen or every decision that might have to be made, so don't try. That's what guidance regarding goals, values, and quality of life are for. Ideally, your surrogate will evaluate treatments and make choices that are consistent with your goals, values, and definitions of quality of life—just as you would have.

Mary, a sixty-nine-year-old woman with mild heart failure, said she had thought a lot about her preferences for care at the end of life. She told me that she would accept intubation but only for forty-eight hours, at which point she would want it disconnected. I asked her what she would want us to do if at forty-eight hours she was still very sick, but we thought that if we waited another forty-eight hours, she'd be well enough to breathe on her own and recover. Not surprisingly, she quickly said, "Well, sure, that would be fine." I then asked how she came to the forty-eight-hour limit and what was important to her about it. She told me that her friend had been trapped for weeks on a ventilator, and she wanted to avoid that fate. She figured forty-eight hours was long enough to know if she would get better. She didn't want to be a prisoner of the ventilator, and interacting with her family and friends was her primary goal.

In the end, she agreed to intubation, provided we thought it would give her a reasonable chance of being awake and able to talk and interact meaningfully. If it was meaningful, she said, she would say so. If she couldn't tell us that it was meaningful, we should assume that it wasn't. And if it took a week or more to figure that out, that was acceptable. Her specificity really helped us.

If you need guidance in choosing and talking with your surrogate and sharing your preferences, visit the PREPARE website (www.prepareforyourcare.org). PREPARE was developed by my good friend and colleague Dr. Rebecca Sudore, a professor at UCSF. PREPARE includes videos that take you through the process step by step. The conversations with your surrogate and your doctor will also help you clarify what is important to you. We think of these conversations as you telling someone what is most important, but many times it's through these conversations that important issues become clear. That's all the more reason to choose a surrogate you trust and whom you can talk to.

CODE STATUS: CPR TO DNR

Another decision that you will be repeatedly asked to make concerns CPR. First, let me explain CPR. Basically, CPR (cardiopulmonary resuscitation) is a procedure that is done to *try* to revive people who have just died. Dying means that their heart stopped and they're no longer breathing. CPR rarely works, because it's really hard to revive someone who has died.

CPR, which is good to learn (see the American Heart Association: www.heart.org), can be provided by anyone who has been trained to give it. It involves pushing on the chest to compress the heart and get blood circulating, mouth-to-mouth breathing, and calling for help. In the hospital or when done by paramedics, the procedure is a bit more involved and includes intubation, electrically shocking the heart to try and get it to beat normally again, and giving medications. You've probably seen it on TV or in movies, which I'll talk more about in a bit.

CPR is the only medical intervention you'll receive without consent unless you specify to the contrary beforehand. All other treatments, even those as simple as blood tests or giving aspirin, require your consent. Decisions about CPR are the sole exception to the rule to focus on goals, not treatments. Whether you want to receive CPR is a vital question that you need to consider.

In the hospital, your preference about whether to undergo CPR is called your "code status." When a patient needs CPR, many hospitals call it a "code blue." You may have heard code blue announcements in a hospital. If you decide that you want to receive CPR in the event you die, it's called a "full code." If you don't want it, then it's a "no code." No code may also be referred to as "do not resuscitate," or DNR. Some hospitals use the wording "do not *attempt* resuscitation" (DNAR) to acknowledge that we try, but don't usually succeed at, resuscitation.

The challenge is that many people, doctors and nurses included, think that no code and DNR mean "do nothing"—that is, don't do anything to help patients live longer—which is simply not true. In reality, no code and DNR only mean that if you die suddenly, we won't try to revive you. The designation doesn't mean anything more. It also doesn't tell us anything about your preferences for any other treatments. And we can do plenty short of CPR to help you feel better and live longer. For example, you can have DNR status and receive chemotherapy.

Do you want CPR? If you are healthy and you have a heart attack or are in a car accident, CPR could give you back your life. But if you have an advanced serious illness such as cancer, heart failure, emphysema, or dementia, CPR isn't likely to help you and could make your condition worse.

My good friend Dr. James Tulsky did a very clever study [11.2] in which he and his colleagues watched three medical shows—*Chicago Hope, Rescue 911*, and *ER*—for one year and noted every time a patient had CPR. They also kept track of whether the CPR worked. On these TV shows, 75 percent of those given CPR survived, and two-thirds of those who survived did well. In real life, about a third of those who receive CPR in a hospital survive, and only about a third of those patients ultimately leave the hospital. The numbers are much worse for CPR that is not performed in hospitals. And in certain situations—for instance, for someone with metastatic cancer—the statistics are much worse.

Receiving CPR means you've died. Even if you survive, you may be much worse off, much sicker than where you started. CPR is not like pushing the reset button on your computer or smartphone, and it's not like jump-starting your car battery.

Ask your doctor what your chances are of being in the 12 percent who leave the hospital after CPR. Push for a real answer. Tell your doctor that it's fine if he has to look it up. Also ask for a recommendation. Knowing you and your medical situation, would your doctor recommend CPR for you?

One more point about CPR: in hospitals, CPR is done by a team of doctors, nurses, pharmacists, respiratory therapists, and others. Controlled chaos fills the room. Different members of the medical team are doing chest compressions, attempting intubation, giving medications, and drawing blood. They create a flurry of activity. Increasingly, family members are being allowed to stay and watch. The scene is scary and shocking if you're not used to it. It is disturbing even to those of us who have been through many codes.

So should you have CPR? In general, for people with advanced illness I would recommend against it. If your illness makes you so sick that your heart stops and you stop breathing, it's your time. CPR isn't likely to work. You have maybe one chance in 200. But more important, if it works, you'll be sicker and worse off. You'll be intubated and in the ICU. You'll still have whatever serious illness caused you to die and need CPR, and now you'll have more complications.

If, despite CPR, you die, your final moments will have been spent at the center of a tornado, and while a team works on your body, your family may be watching with horror or be banished from the room. In either case, they won't be with you, at your side, holding your hand.

Many seriously ill patients I talk to about CPR initially say, "Sure, why not? What have I got to lose?" CPR is not risk-free—for you or your loved ones. Most people die once. Think about how you want that to be for you and how you want your loved ones to remember it. Don't choose to have CPR because of some fantasy that it will make you better or keep you alive. It can be hard on your family members as well. CPR can't make you better and may only serve to keep you alive in a way you don't want.

Don't worry that saying no to CPR is saying no to the many other things that we can do to help you feel better and live longer. I recommend that my seriously ill patients let go of CPR and focus on the many measures we can take to help them feel better, live longer, and achieve their goals. In chapter 12, I'll discuss what those other measures are.

ADVANCE HEALTH CARE DIRECTIVES

Put your wishes in writing. Leave no doubt as to precisely the kind of care you want and the quality of life that is acceptable to you. Expressing your wishes in writing will make your preferences clear and increase the chances that they'll be followed.

The legal name for instructions regarding your health care is advance health care directives. Advance health care directives are legal documents that fall into two categories: (1) living wills and (2) durable power of attorney for health care, which is also called a health care proxy. You must be at least eighteen years old to execute these directives.

> **NOTE:** Advance health care directives are binding legal documents that are governed by state law, and they can differ from state to state. All directives must be written, signed, and witnessed and/or notarized.
>
> This chapter is intended to give you basic information about advance health care directives, not legal advice. Its purpose is to inform you of the existence of advance health care directives, briefly describe them, and emphasize their importance. Check the requirements in your state.

A living will states your wishes regarding life-sustaining medical treatment if you're terminally ill, permanently unconscious, or in the end stage of a fatal illness. A living will essentially says that if you have a terminal illness and are dying, you instruct your physicians to let you die. Living wills are preferable to no written instructions, but they are more limited than a durable power of attorney for health care. I strongly recommend that you complete an advance directive and that when you do, you make it a durable power of attorney for health care.

A durable power of attorney for health care enables you to name a surrogate to make decisions on your behalf if you can't make them yourself. In a durable power of attorney for health care, you can also include the values, preferences, and quality of life you want to guide decisions.

Like any legal document, you must be competent when you sign an advance health care directive. Many people worry that when they sign a legal document it can't be changed. However, you can always change an advance directive. It is not uncommon for people to change their preferences over time, especially as their illness progresses. You can change your surrogate and your preferences, and you can complete a new, updated durable power of attorney for health care, though changing often will add confusion, not clarity. Be sure to update your surrogate as your thoughts evolve.

Let your family members, legal, health, or other appropriate professionals know that you have an advance health care directive and what it says. Give copies to them. Don't put it in a safe or a safe deposit box—you want it to be easily accessible when you need it. Some people put it on the fridge, some in a desk drawer. Choose a safe, easily accessible place for your advance directive and tell people where it is.

In addition to giving copies to your surrogate and family members, give your doctor a copy and bring one to the hospital every time. I have a file folder in my office with my patients' advance directives, and I also upload them to our electronic medical record so that all the doctors and nurses in our system have access to them. An advance directive won't do you any good unless it is available when needed, so make sure yours is readily available.

Discussing your wishes with your family can be delicate, so expect resistance. Sit down with them at a time and place where you all can be relaxed. Assess their moods and receptivity. If they seem reluctant, don't throw everything at them at once. Simply tell them that you have an advance health care directive, where it is, and briefly what it says. Save the details for a later time.

PHYSICIAN ORDERS FOR LIFE-SUSTAINNING TREATMENT (POLST)

An advance directive, which should be filled out by every adult regardless of their health status, provides a broad outline of your wishes relating to your end-of-life care. When you're seriously ill, you should also complete a physician orders for life-sustaining treatment (POLST) form, which documents your preferences for *specific* treatments and has the force of a physician order.

Developed in Oregon two decades ago, POLST is a standardized medical order form that complements, but does not replace, an advance health care directive and indicates your preferences regarding three specific issues: (1) CPR, (2) medical treatments that can range from all treatments to those focused solely on comfort, and (3) artificial nutrition and feeding tubes. This form is signed by you or your surrogate and your doctor and is designed to travel with a patient across medical settings.

According to the CHCF survey [11.1], nearly two-thirds of Californians would want to complete a POLST form if they became seriously ill, including 77 percent of those who were sixty-five or older. Seventy-one percent said they would want a seriously ill loved one to complete the form so they could understand their wishes.

The power of the POLST form comes from the fact that, as its name states, it is a physician order. A POLST form enshrines your wishes as a physician order that paramedics and emergency room doctors and nurses can follow. For more information about POLST and to see if your state uses it, visit www.polst.org. Some states use different names for the same purpose: MOLST (medical orders for life-sustaining treatments), MOST (medical orders for scope of treatment), and POST (physician order for scope of treatment).

STATE TO STATE

Laws on advance health care directives exist in all states, but the requirements, terminology, and names differ from state to state. For example, some states require a second doctor to certify your doctor's finding that you are incapable of making treatment decisions before your surrogate can refuse life-sustaining medical treatments on your behalf. Check the laws in your state.

Advance health care directives executed in one state may be accepted in other states. Usually, directives will be honored by states that have similar requirements. However, the opposite may also be true: out-of-state directives may not be honored.

The ultimate goal of an advance health care directive is to ensure that your goals, values, and preferences guide your care even if you're not able to express them in the moment. To that end, a written, signed, witnessed document is strong evidence of what your wishes are, and it should be respected by doctors and nurses even if the form is slightly different than the one used in their state. Nonetheless, if you spend time in more than one state, execute separate advance health care directives for each state, even though their requirements may be the same or similar. It can help avoid problems down the line.

> You can find advance directive documents online. You can also get them at your doctor's office and the hospital. Because different states have specific rules about advance directives, check websites for your state medical board or state hospital association, or simply search "*(your state name) advance directive*" online to find documents you can use. Excellent and easy-to-use advance directives can be found at the following sites:
> www.iha4health.org/our-services/advance-directive/
> www.agingwithdignity.org/five-wishes/about-five-wishes

You don't need a lawyer to complete an advance health care directive. Most states have easy-to-follow forms that you can download from the Internet. You simply fill in the blanks and have it witnessed and/or notarized at the time you sign it. Advance health care directive forms usually provide room for you to include additional wishes and directions and instructions about organ donations, burial, and cremation.

RX

Every adult should have an advance health care directive regardless of his or her age. Younger people tend to think that they don't need one yet, that they have plenty of time. However, the future is uncertain and unpredictable. Accidents occur, serious illnesses come on suddenly, and you can become incapacitated. So be prepared: complete an advance health care directive.

Talking with your loved ones about your preferences and goals can be difficult. Your loved ones may be in denial and want to avoid these difficult conversations. Tell them that you're doing this out of love for them so that they're not burdened by making decisions on your behalf or left feeling guilty about those they make. Remind them that avoiding the conversation doesn't mean that they won't have to make decisions about your care—it only means that they will be unprepared.

I've seen too many people receive care they didn't want and family members agonizing over decisions that could have been anticipated or for which guidance could have been given. Completing an advance health care directive and appointing a surrogate are not a total guarantee that everything will go smoothly, but no better way exists for putting the odds in your favor. Don't be another statistic, an example of a patient and family that didn't talk.

chapter twelve

PALLIATIVE CARE: YOU MAY NOT KNOW WHAT IT MEANS, BUT YOU WANT IT

I'M OFTEN CALLED IN TO TALK TO SERIOUSLY ILL PATIENTS about palliative care. When I introduce myself and say that I'm a palliative care doctor, I usually get little or no response, only blank stares. While more and more people say that they have heard the term, most patients I meet don't know what palliative care is. Some think that it's hospice care, which is half right and half wrong because all hospice care is palliative care, but all palliative care isn't hospice care. I'll say more about this point later in this chapter.

Numerous studies show that *people with serious illness and their loved ones live longer and better with palliative care*. If palliative care were a pill, every doctor would prescribe it and every seriously ill person would take it [12.1].

I continually see the benefits of palliative care. When I initially meet patients, I explain that palliative care is a distinct medical specialty that helps seriously ill people live as well as possible for as long as possible and helps relieve their pain, stress, and other symptoms. The blank stares vanish, and they reply, "That sounds great. I want it."

The main reason that patients don't know about palliative care is that it's a relatively new medical specialty, and it focuses on a particular segment of the population: the seriously ill. Since most people avoid conversations about serious illness, awareness of palliative care and its benefits doesn't usually filter down to most of them.

The term "palliative care" also doesn't help. It's confusing and certainly not descriptive or informative. I constantly have to explain its meaning. Put simply, palliative care is *medical care focused on improving quality of life for people with serious illness*. When the term is used, people frequently say, "Boy, that's a bad name," but when I tell them what it is, they're all in. Almost every seriously ill patient wants it, and their loved ones want it for them.

Those who tell me they've heard of palliative care generally misunderstand it. Palliative care is riddled by misconceptions, myths, and erroneous information, which I'll clear up in a bit. The most important misconception is that people think palliative care is about dying, which isn't surprising given that many doctors and nurses also make the same mistake.

An important message I want to share is that palliative care is *not* about dying, but *is* about living well with serious illness. It's available to patients at any stage of any serious illness such as cancer, heart failure, lung disease, chronic liver disease, emphysema, kidney failure, ALS, Parkinson's disease, dementia, and stroke. If you or someone you care about is seriously ill, getting palliative care is one of the best things you or they can do.

The danger with thinking that palliative care is only about dying is that you may wait until you're about to die before you seek palliative care. That's way too late. Although palliative care will help when you're dying, getting it sooner will help you more. Another important point is that you don't have to choose between palliative care and any other type of care for your serious illness. You can and should get both at the same time! If you wait to get palliative care, you'll miss out on all the benefits that palliative care could have provided to help you live better and longer.

Palliative care helps patients and their loved ones deal with the issues that are of the greatest concern to people with serious illness:

> *Relief from distressing symptoms:* Palliative care focuses on alleviating patients' symptoms, including their pain, fatigue, shortness of breath, anxiety, nausea, and depression. Palliative care team members are experts at providing symptom relief.

> *Clear communication and decision making:* In chapters 10 and 11, I talked about how to determine what is most important to you and letting that guide your care. Palliative care is provided by teams that excel in helping you explore, clarify, and express your values and goals and how you define quality of life. They help you review your treatment options and make good decisions that are consistent with your values, beliefs, and what is most important to you. Team members conduct ongoing conversations with patients to help them understand and articulate their feelings, develop good treatment plans, and document those preferences in advance health care directives.

> *Support:* Palliative care teams provide emotional, spiritual, and practical support. In the field, we call it "psycho-social-spiritual support." Social workers help with emotional support and practical concerns such as where patients will

be cared for, how they will be cared for, who will care for them, and financial issues. Practical concerns can be extremely stressful. Despite the impact of these factors on patients' quality of life, traditional care frequently doesn't clearly and explicitly deal with them—but palliative care does. Chaplains and spiritual care providers help with spiritual needs, which may include and go beyond religious issues and rituals to questions about meaning, relationships, and legacy. (I discuss these in more detail in chapters 10 and 14.) At the core of palliative care is a focus on the patient *and* the family, and palliative care benefits family members as well as patients. For example, the survivors of patients who received palliative care have less depression [12.2].

> ## YOU'RE THE EXPERT ABOUT YOU
>
> Talking with patients about their values, goals, and definitions of quality of life is one of the most important parts of my work as a palliative care physician. I come to each conversation openly, with no set idea or agenda as to what may be best. My goal is always to deeply and honestly understand each person's values and goals, to truly know what they hope for, and to help them get care that will allow them to achieve their goals. My only agenda is to hear what my patients consider most important, to share what I know about the options that could help them achieve their goals, and to help them make the best possible decision.
>
> In the end, no one knows better than you, the patient, what is right or best for you. Not family members, not friends, not a surrogate, and not doctors or nurses. Sure, we all have ideas and opinions. And we can share them. But you are the ultimate authority about what is best for you.

EXTRA LAYER OF SUPPORT

No one person in health care is an expert in all the issues patients with serious illness and their families face. It takes a group of clinicians to address all the key aspects of care, and that is why palliative care is provided by a *team* of doctors, nurses, social workers, chaplains, and others, including physical therapists and pharmacists. Team members are specialists with expertise in the broad range of important issues faced by patients with serious illness.

Palliative care teams don't replace your medical team but rather work with your other doctors and nurses to provide you with "an extra layer of support," as the Center to Advance Palliative Care (www.capc.org) calls it. When dealing with serious illness, everyone can use more support.

Working together as a team offers insights into issues that might be vague or unclear to any individual team member and the patient.

During an examination, I asked Victor, a young patient who was dying from cystic fibrosis, "When you look to the future, what do you hope will happen?" He replied, "I'm really trying to figure out what God's plan is for me."

Victor's answer threw me, and I didn't know how to respond or exactly what he meant. So I discussed it with our team's chaplain, Denah Joseph, who is an ordained Buddhist chaplain. She had had several long conversations with Victor, during which he talked about his spirituality. Denah told me, "I think what Victor was trying to say is that he feels the treatments aren't helping him anymore, and he probably wants to stop them. He also doesn't want to be intubated again. But if he made that decision, it would be difficult for his family to hear. They would see it as giving up and going against God. So Victor expressed it in terms of what God wants him to do because if God says it's OK to decide against more treatments, it would be more acceptable to his family.

Denah's insight was invaluable. It opened up a whole new area of exploration for us, an area that I was unaware of and probably never would have discovered on my own. By focusing on Victor's spirituality and his concern for his family, we were able to help reduce his stress so he could be more comfortable and at ease. Then we asked him, "What do you think God wants for you? How do you think your family will react if you stop your treatments?"

Working together as a team, we were able to help Victor achieve the goals that were most important to him. He was able to respect his family and address his own pain and discomfort with a clear, guilt-free conscience. The team approach helped us to see issues that any one of us alone would have missed. That insight helped us open up doors that we otherwise wouldn't have known existed.

Palliative care team members are experts at helping patients clarify and express their wishes and goals. For example, during conversations with a palliative care team, patients often reveal that they want to go home. They may not come right out and say it because they don't want to burden their families. Team members know how to spot patients' concerns and then discuss them with those patients so they can work together to find viable solutions.

Fulfilling patients' wishes isn't always easy. When you're seriously ill, special arrangements may be required. Arrangements may have to be made to get the right home care, to create the best environment, to get equipment and medications, and to bring all necessary services together.

Often, patients have unusual requests, and arranging for them takes special understanding, experience, talent, relationships, and resourcefulness.

Bobby's situation was grave. He was bedridden in the ICU and the end was near. At twenty-eight, Bobby had stomach cancer, was on a large dose of pain medication, couldn't eat, was getting intravenous nutrition, and had a tube draining his stomach. He hated being in the ICU and the thought of dying there. Bobby wanted to leave the hospital and spend his remaining days at his friend's house, which was an hour-and-a-half drive from the hospital through a maze of steep, narrow, winding roads. His friends were all for it and agreed to take shifts caring for him. Bobby's plan was to go to the house and stop his intravenous nutrition after three days. He wanted to spend his remaining time looking out through the trees, across the valley, and to the sea.

I loved Bobby's plan, but I had no idea how to implement it. The house was an hour away from the nearest medical facility, and there were countless details to work out. This was no cookie-cutter discharge. However, Jane Hawgood, our palliative care team's social worker, knew exactly what to do. With no time to lose, she promptly made all the arrangements. Jane found an ambulance company that would agree to make the difficult trip to the house. She then identified a company that would deliver all the equipment and medicines. Jane also arranged for a hospice agency to provide nurses to stay with Bobby onsite and manage all the complex equipment and machines—something that is not typically done. Jane had worked closely with this hospice for years;

she trusted them, they trusted her, and together they were able to quickly create a workable plan.

Although complications arose, including a blocked tube, the hospice nurse was able to fix them, and everything else went smoothly. Thanks to Jane, Bobby got his wish. His final days were spent peacefully with friends.

> Just a few years ago, palliative care was hard to find outside of hospices. As we go to press, it's currently provided in more than 1,600 hospitals in the United States, according to the Center to Advance Palliative Care. Approximately 67 percent of hospitals with more than fifty beds now have a palliative care team, and over 90 percent of large hospitals offer palliative care. If you or your loved one has a serious illness and is hospitalized, ask for palliative care.
>
> Medicare, Medicaid, and all health insurance companies cover palliative care. If your doctor says you don't need it or are not ready for it, politely but firmly disagree and demand palliative care. The palliative care team will help you feel better.

PROVEN BENEFIT

The Internet is abuzz with all sorts of claims of the latest cure for a serious illness. Every time you turn around, the wonders of some new cure or treatment are being promoted. Sadly, few of those claims have been proven. They haven't been rigorously studied, and the alleged benefits have never been confirmed.

In contrast, the benefits of palliative care are well documented. They've been studied, and research has shown that palliative care helps patients with serious illness and their survivors.

Palliative care helps seriously ill patients in hospitals, in clinics, and via hospice services.

The evidence proving palliative care's benefits is clear and overwhelming. Studies have found that:

> People who receive palliative care *live longer and have a better quality of life* with less pain and depression [12.3].

> Palliative care patients are less likely to spend time in an ICU near the end of life [12.4].

> After patients who received palliative care die, their loved ones fare better than survivors of those who didn't get palliative care. Survivors of those who got palliative care have less depression and are less likely to die within the next year [12.5, 12.6].

> Palliative care isn't harmful. To be precise, no study has found any evidence that palliative care causes harm. That can't be said of chemotherapy, surgery, transplants, and other treatments, many of which cause wounds, scars, pain, discomfort, and other harmful side effects. Palliative care has no bad side effects. The American Society of Clinical Oncology, the world's largest cancer doctor organization, published a provisional clinical opinion recommending palliative care to oncologists [12.7]. This guide stated that "substantial evidence demonstrates that palliative care—when combined with standard cancer care or as the main focus of care—leads to better patient and caregiver outcomes [including] improvement in symptoms, quality of life, and patient satisfaction, with reduced caregiver burden." The guide went on to recommend palliative care for patients who have metastatic cancer of any kind. This endorsement is based on evidence from many studies that show that palliative care helps [12.7].

To learn more about palliative care, watch these videos, which are from a course we put on for the public at UCSF:

www.uctv.tv/shows/Palliative-Care-Who-is-it-For-What-Does-it-Do-Why-Should-I-Want-it-and-When-29714

www.uctv.tv/palliative-care

WHOLE PERSON CARE

Much is written today about precision medicine. The idea is to target treatments precisely to your illness—for example, determining the genetic defect in your cancer cells and selecting a chemotherapy agent that hits that very mutation. Some of these treatments hold great promise. Maybe one day they will even help us choose pain medications targeted to your opioid receptors. But even when this approach is useful, it misses the essential point that we are more than our genes and that having our DNA sequenced to find the right medicines for our illness is just one small part of the puzzle. We define health as much more than a biologic event. Wellness and healing focus on the whole person—our emotions, spiritual needs, beliefs, and social environment, which define who we are as much as our genes do.

Palliative care provides whole person care, and the team addresses all facets of who you are as a person. Palliative care is the ultimate in precision medicine, with treatments targeted precisely to who you are as a person. Palliative care integrates all the latest treatments, such as heart pumps, immunotherapy for cancer, and genetic testing, as well as emotional and spiritual care to heal every part of you.

In treating the whole person, innumerable nonmedical factors come into play. They include:

> Who you are in your family—a grandfather, grandmother, father, mother, uncle, aunt, son, or daughter.
> Who you are in your community—a boss, partner, employee, doctor, engineer, salesperson, politician, coach, scout leader, or library volunteer.
> How you see yourself.
> What roles are important to you. Are you too sick to fulfill those roles? How can you continue to fulfill all or some of those roles? What accommodations will be needed?
> What your illness means for you, your family, your relationships, your business or career, your community, and your legacy.
> How you find meaning in what's happening to you.

In treating patients, palliative care realizes that one size doesn't fit all. So it works to understand each person and personalize his or her care. This is why understanding your goals is so crucial. For instance, in treating pain, palliative care teams tailor the regimen of pain medications to the individual to achieve the right balance between pain control and alertness. If a medicine doesn't work or causes unpleasant or harmful side effects, the dosage can be adjusted, it can be used in combination with other medications, or a different medication can be prescribed. In the process, palliative care teams closely monitor each patient. They assess treatments, look for side effects, and see what is working and what isn't.

Close communications, and maintaining an ongoing dialogue with patients, is a central feature of palliative care. Throughout patients' treatment, teams continually conduct "palliative care conversations"; they talk with patients so that both they and the patients can discover what patients' goals are and what treatments are most likely to help them achieve them. Palliative care teams and patients form partnerships to understand each patient's values, beliefs, and priorities. In these conversations, patients reveal vital information that they otherwise might not disclose. Often, this information enables them to make more of the time they have left.

Team members are experts in communication and trained to ask incisive questions, listen, and recognize clues that are subtle but informative. From those clues, team members can probe more deeply and elicit crucial information from patients. When they disclose that information, patients come to realizations that they may have ignored, suppressed, or not understood. Often, patients express their fears, which team members help them work through. Palliative care conversations help patients come to understandings about themselves and their priorities.

RELIEVING STRESS

Palliative care teams focus on relieving the stress of serious illness. They know that being seriously ill is extremely stressful. It's also stressful for patients' families and friends. Stress is debilitating: it wears you down and tends to make illnesses worse. Anyone who has ever been sick or had a loved one or close friend who was sick knows how much stress illness can cause.

Most traditional approaches for treating serious illness don't focus on stress. Usually, they deal with the biological factors and symptoms and don't address the impact that the illness and its symptoms has on patients and their loved ones. Too often, the stress of serious illness is accepted as an unavoidable part of the experience. Doctors and nurses may see stress as inevitable, as something that can't be relieved or reduced. When stress becomes so great that it must be addressed, it's often too late.

From the outset, palliative care teams work to reduce stress for patients and their loved ones. The ongoing conversations between patients and palliative care teams help relieve patients' stress. These conversations are cathartic. Patients find expressing their fears, hopes, and concerns liberating. Opening up and expressing their feelings provides relief. Often, patients can be more open and forthright with palliative care team members than they can be with others, including their family and friends. When patients talk with palliative care team members, they can understand themselves better.

When patients discuss their stress with a palliative care team, it can lead to solutions that reduce their stress. They may worry about where they will live, who will care for them, or no longer being a breadwinner or caretaker. They may fear a future with pain or dependence on others. When you know what the issues are, many of them can be handled. Although some causes of stress, such as financial pressures, may not go away, talking about them can be beneficial.

WHO NEEDS PALLIATIVE CARE AND WHEN

As you read this chapter, you may wonder if you need palliative care and, if so, when and where to get it. If you or your loved one is seriously ill—if you have one of the following conditions—you need palliative care now.

> Metastatic cancer
> Heart failure that required you to be hospitalized more than once in a year

> Emphysema or another lung disease that required you to be hospitalized more than once in a year
> ALS (Lou Gehrig's disease)
> Kidney failure that requires dialysis
> Cirrhosis
> Liver, heart, or lung failure and are on a waiting list for a transplant
> Leukemia, myeloma, or lymphoma and are undergoing a bone marrow transplant or your disease has relapsed after initial treatment
> A debilitating stroke that has left you impaired or weak
> Dementia and are having difficulty caring for yourself
> Advanced Parkinson's or Huntington's disease
> Many chronic illnesses that taken together make it hard for you to care for yourself and force you to stay close to home

The current approach to palliative care shows that it should be started at the time of diagnosis and be provided alongside any disease-focused treatments for your serious illness. (See Figure 12.1.) Over time, as you get sicker, you likely will want and need more palliative care. The approach shows that you don't have to choose between disease-focused treatments and palliative care: throughout the course of your illness, you can get both. The figure also shows that care for the bereaved family members is also an important part of care and that the sense of grief and loss lasts forever, though it does get less intense. This approach to care helps people with serious illness *live as well as possible for as long as possible.*

Finding palliative care can be challenging. Palliative care is a relatively new field, and programs are still being developed. You can find palliative care programs in your area by visiting www.getpalliativecare.org. Also contact your doctor or your lo-

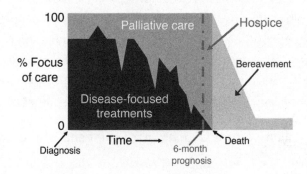

FIGURE 12.1

Current approach to palliative care
alongside any treatment for your illness

"Live as well as possible for as long as possible"

cal hospital, or search its website for "palliative care," "support-ive care," or "symptom management." Some palliative care teams use these other names because doctors tell them that they would be more likely to refer patients if they use a name other than palliative care. In our program at UCSF, we use "palliative care" and "symptom management" to appeal to as many people as possible. In the end, the name is not important. The care is.

Call hospice agencies. More and more hospice agencies now offer palliative care that is separate from hospice care. Or simply search "palliative care" and "[your city or area]."

THE TRUTH ABOUT PALLIATIVE CARE: DEBUNKING MYTHS

Palliative care is greatly misunderstood by patients and health care providers. When I speak to groups, I'm usually asked ques-tions that reveal common myths and misconceptions that may keep people from getting palliative care. You may have many of these questions, so let me clarify the ones that are most common.

Truth: You don't have to choose between living well and living long.

The studies are clear: With palliative care, you can live longer *and* better. You don't have to choose; you can have both. Studies also confirm that palliative care helps seriously ill people have a better quality of life with less pain and depression, and it reduces the chance that patients' loved ones will experience depression or complicated grief after the patients die. Get palliative care along with any other treatment for your serious illness.

Truth: Palliative care is much more than end-of-life care.

Palliative care *is* for people approaching the end of life, but it isn't *only* for those at the end of life. Palliative care is right for people at all stages of serious illness. You can, and should, get palliative care along with curative care at any stage of your illness. Put another way, all end-of-life care is palliative care, but not all palliative care is end-of-life care. (See Figure 12.2.) If you're seriously ill, seek palliative care promptly. Get it as soon as you can. Start the moment you get your diagnosis. If you're diagnosed with cancer, make an appointment with an oncologist and say, "Please refer me to a palliative care doctor. I want the best care I can get, and I want palliative care on my team."

Doctors and nurses frequently tell their patients, "You're not ready for palliative care." It's a common misperception. Explain to your doctor that you're not giving up and that you want the best care possible. Seeing a palliative care specialist promptly will help you learn what you may be in for and make the best treatment choices. You may not need to see a palliative care team regularly, but you'll learn where to turn when you do, which will save you time and energy if you need them in the future.

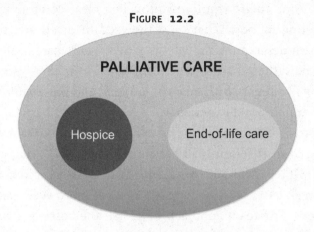

FIGURE 12.2

PALLIATIVE CARE

Hospice

End-of-life care

Truth: Palliative care is not just hospice care.

This is the most common misconception I hear. The fact is that all hospice care and end-of-life care is palliative care, but not all palliative care is hospice or end-of-life care. Hospice, which has been around for a long time, is the most widely available way to receive palliative care, so it's understandable that people have this misconception. In the United States, hospice care is provided to people with serious illness who have six months or less to live, but palliative care is available to you at any stage of your illness. Unlike hospice care, palliative care is given along with curative treatments.

In the United States, specific rules define hospice. I'll explain them in the next chapter and discuss how this wonderful service works and how to make the most of it.

Truth: Palliative care is more than just good medical care that all doctors and nurses should provide.

This statement is basically true, but it's misleading because it doesn't tell the whole story. Without question, all health care providers should focus on improving their patients' quality of life, relieving their symptoms, providing clear communication, and offering support. That's just the good medical care that every patient deserves. Although we expect health care professionals to know these basics, the ability to address these issues for seriously ill patients with nuance, subtlety, and skill requires specialized training and experience.

Palliative care specialists have been rigorously trained and certified to treat seriously ill patients. They're up to date on advances in their field and work with your personal physician to give you an extra layer of support. You get more eyes, ears, and knowhow. The team approach covers all the bases and reduces the chances of important matters being missed.

When you learn that you have a heart condition, you may not immediately need to see a cardiologist or a heart failure specialist. Your primary care physician can usually manage your care. You may, however, decide to see a heart specialist to confirm the diagnosis and chart a course of treatment that the primary care physician can manage. If your heart condition gets worse, you may need to be treated by a specialist who can fine-tune your treatment. The specialist may know of and be able to provide treatments that your primary care physician can't.

The same is true with palliative care. Many issues that a palliative care team addresses can be handled by your doctor—just as your primary care doctor can manage many issues related to heart failure. When you find out that you're seriously ill, you may not need to see a palliative care team right away or regularly, especially early on. However, as your illness progresses, you may want to work with a palliative care team to control your symptoms and get help making treatment decisions. If at the time of diagnosis your illness is very advanced—for example, you have metastatic cancer or require a heart transplant—see a palliative care specialist right away.

Truth: People want to talk about illness and end of life and want palliative care.

When people are well, they don't want to think or talk about being sick. They want to concentrate on staying well. However, as I previously stated, a survey conducted by the California Health Care Foundation [12.8] found that the vast majority of people say that if they were seriously ill, they would like to talk with their doctors about their wishes for medical treatment toward the end of life.

> Whenever I talk with seriously ill people, they're almost always willing to have conversations about their values, hopes, and goals. In fact, most are eager. They react similarly to palliative care. Even though most people don't know about it or what it is, when I explain it, virtually all of them want to talk about it. After our conversation they often tell me that not only do they want palliative care for themselves and their loved ones, but also that it should be a standard part of our health care system.

Seriously ill patients don't usually push to receive palliative care. As I said, many don't know about it, and others tell me, "I'm waiting for my doctor to bring it up." It's important for doctors to raise the subject, and it's equally important for patients and their loved ones to initiate conversations about palliative care with their doctors. If you want palliative care, which you should, ask for it and don't take no for an answer.

Truth: Palliative care is about more than helping you have a good death.

I've cared for thousands of seriously ill people and have been with many of them as they died, but I've never seen a good death, and

I don't believe that it exists. Simply put, there is no good death. The truth is that the end of life is filled with loss, sadness, and grief, none of which are good. Some deaths are more peaceful, humane, dignified, pain free, and comfortable than others, and I do my best to make them so. I have no doubt that this kind of death is better than a death filled with pain, chaos, and discomfort. Too often the medical care provided makes things worse and only adds to patients' pain, discomfort, and loss of dignity.

Even when we're able to help patients be at peace, be dignified, and be pain free, death is still not good. I can't imagine a death so good that people line up for it. Quite the opposite, people embrace life and want to live it as well and as long as possible. I'm not in the business of good death—I'm in the business of good life.

The focus of palliative care is not on death, but on life. It's on helping you live as well as possible for as long as possible. Palliative care can help make the end of life more comfortable and peaceful, but its greatest benefit is in helping you live well and long. It does so by helping you understand your goals and determining what treatments can help you achieve them.

RX

As a palliative care specialist, my goal is, first and foremost, to help you have a good, long life, and, second, when the end inevitably comes, to make the end of your life as dignified and comfortable as it can be. Since we all have our own ways of approaching illness and the end of life, I'm not judgmental; I don't try to tell you how your life and death should be. Instead, I try to help you express and understand your values and wishes and get care that is consistent with them. I want to ensure that the treatments you choose help more than hurt and don't undermine your most important goals. My role is not to prescribe how your life and death should proceed, but to help you make the most of every moment and help you have as many moments as possible. That's what this book is about—making the most of your life in the face of serious illness.

It's really quite simple: palliative care helps you get through serious illness. It enables you to live as well as possible for as long as possible, to make the most of your remaining time. Palliative care lets you have the best possible quality of life as *you* define it.

As you deal with your illness, get palliative care! Serious illness is multilayered and complex. Choosing treatments and making decisions is hard and can be bewildering. It takes a team of experts to help you make the best decisions and get the best care. The specialists on palliative care teams are experts who are not invested in a particular treatment. They're dedicated to helping you weigh your options carefully and objectively, helping you choose treatments wisely, and helping you live as well as possible for as long as possible.

chapter thirteen

HOSPICE CARE

HOSPICE CARE IS A HUMANE AND COMPASSIONATE SER-vice for people who have been diagnosed to have six months or less to live. Its mission is to help patients live well with serious illness and have comfort and dignity at the end of their lives. Hospice care focuses on controlling patients' pain and symptoms, but it does not attempt to cure their illnesses or postpone their deaths. As I've mentioned, all hospice care is palliative care. And hospice is not a one-way street. You can enroll in hospice, and if you later decide to pursue curative treatments, you can disenroll from hospice and re-enroll later. About 15 percent of people disenroll, or "graduate," from hospice.

Many people think of hospice as a place, and in other parts of the world it is. In the United States, hospice is a service that is generally provided at home; however, residential hospice facilities also exist. Hospice is also a philosophy of care tailored to each patient's needs. Like all good palliative care, hospice care assists patients and their loved ones as they go through these difficult times. Hospice helps patients and their families shift their focus from the illness to optimizing the quality of the time they have to spend together.

Hospice care, like all palliative care, is provided by teams. Typically, a team consists of the patient's personal physician, the hospice physician, nurses, home health aides, therapists, social workers, chaplains, and volunteers. The hospice team works closely with your personal physician to coordinate your care and serves as your physician's eyes and ears. Hospice team members visit you at home as often as necessary but are not round-the-clock caregivers. Team members are available 24/7 by phone, and hospice nurses and doctors will come to your home in emergencies.

Hospice teams provide numerous services based on the patient's and his or her family's needs and wishes. They coach families on how to care for their loved ones. Hospices also provide pain control and emotional support and furnish medications for hospice-qualifying conditions, supplies, and equipment such as hospital beds, oxygen, suction, and bedside commodes. In addition, teams perform and arrange for other needed services, including speech, memory, physical, and occupational therapies and getting patients the spiritual support they need and want. Hospice volunteers can also assist with household tasks, run errands, and make appointments.

While my grandfather was receiving in-home hospice care, he wanted a haircut. At eighty-six years old, he still had a full head of hair. He was meticulous about his appearance and felt he was getting a bit shaggy. Since he was bedbound, we weren't sure we could get him out for a haircut. My aunt mentioned it to the hospice nurse and, as it turned out, one of the hospice volunteers was a barber. He came to my grandparents' apartment and gave my grandfather a haircut. "One of the best I ever had!" my Saba said.

While most people receive hospice care in their homes, hospice care is also provided in in-patient hospice facilities, nursing homes, long-term care facilities, and hospitals. When patients receive hospice care, their curative treatments like chemotherapy are stopped, but medicines to manage their serious illness—for example, for heart failure or Parkinson's disease—continue.

Hospice workers can provide much-needed breaks for caregivers. These breaks, which are called respites, can be for a few hours to a few days. When they're for days, or if symptoms such as pain can't be controlled quickly at home, patients can be admitted to a facility such as a nursing home or hospital.

Some hospice patients improve to the point where they no longer need hospice care, so those services are stopped. We like to say they "graduated" from hospice because they became too well to be eligible for hospice care even though they may have wanted to continue it. Some hospices will stay in touch with patients after "graduation" to make sure that they're doing well. They can re-enroll in hospice whenever they have the need.

Patients can also decide to stop receiving hospice care at any time. Patients who decide to stop hospice care are typically still eligible to receive it. To stop care, they're required to sign a form that gives the date that their hospice care will end. If, however, they subsequently need hospice care, they can receive it again.

Although enrolling in hospice care is often presented as a major decision and a big transition, you don't really have to be ready for anything with hospice except to receive really good care at home and be willing, for the moment, to stop taking disease-focused treatments. That's it.

ELIGIBILITY AND RULES

Hospice care is covered by just about every health care payer, including Medicare and Medicaid. It's available to patients of any age. To enroll in hospice, the patient's doctor and the hospice medical director must sign a statement that the patient has a life-limiting serious illness and a life expectancy of six months or less if the illness runs its usual course. The patient must also sign a statement verifying that he or she is choosing hospice care.

Hospice services will provide these statements for you and your doctor. The six-month prognosis rule doesn't mean that you're automatically discharged from hospice at that point. Hospice services can, and do, continue for more than six months, and it's wonderful when patients live longer. The only requirement for hospice services to continue is that the hospice physician must recertify that the patient is continuing to decline.

For most insurers, including Medicare, enrolling in hospice means that you agree that hospice will provide your medical care. Hospice is not for people who want all the curative medical interventions they can get. It's for those who decide that they want to focus on their comfort and not pursue curative treatments—for now. You can still see your doctor in the office, or at home if she makes house calls, but in general, hospitalizations, emergency room visits, radiation, chemotherapy, and operations are not part of hospice treatment plans.

In exchange, you get more services at home and an entire team to help care for you, and your medications for your serious illness are covered. Unlike patients who receive home health care, if you're enrolled in hospice, you don't have to be home-bound. You can leave your home and even travel, in which case your hospice will contact a hospice in the community you visit to provide care if needed.

FINDING A HOSPICE

In the United States, hospice care is provided by over 6,100 organizations. Unlike palliative care, which is mainly provided in hospitals and just starting to be available outside of hospitals, hospice services are available in virtually every community in the country. The best way to find a hospice is through your personal physician or your hospital's discharge personnel. Since many communities have more than one hospice, you might want to speak with people whose loved ones have had hospice care to find the hospice that would be best for you.

You can learn more about hospice and find a local hospice at the website of the National Hospice and Palliative Care Organization (NHPCO; www.nhpco.org/about/hospice-care). Other organizations, such as the American Cancer Society, United Way, and Visiting Nurses Associations, may also be helpful. To find a hospice, you can also search the word *hospice* and the name of your community on the Internet and even locate local hospices under the word *hospice* on Google Maps.

THE SOONER, THE BETTER

In 2014, the most recent year for which we have data, about 45 percent of Americans who died used hospice services [13.1] (see www.nhpco.org/hospice-statistics-research-press-room/facts -hospice-and-palliative-care). Over the years, that number has steadily increased. When I began my career, only 15 percent of Americans who died made use of hospice. Unfortunately, while more people are now using hospice, they're using it for shorter periods of time.

The median length of time that patients receive hospice care is seventeen days. Although your doctor must certify that your prognosis is six months or less in order for you to qualify for hospice services, half of all hospice patients are referred late in their illnesses and end up receiving less than seventeen days of hospice care. Overall, 35 percent of patients are referred to hospice so late in their illnesses that they receive hospice for less than seven days, and only 10 percent get it for more than six months.

Short courses of hospice care are unfortunate because longer periods of hospice care are associated with better quality of life. In a study of seriously ill patients with cancer, quality of life near the end of life was increased the longer the patient was enrolled in hospice [13.2]. Quality of life at the end of life for those who receive hospice care for a week or less was the same as for those who got no hospice care and much lower than that reported by those who received hospice care for more than a week.

HAVE YOUR CAKE AND EAT IT

I believe that a major reason the duration of hospice care is so short is an unintended consequence of how hospices are paid. Hospices receive a daily rate that has to cover all treatments and medications for your serious illness, as well as all the equipment you need and the entire hospice team. Many treatments that are palliative (which in this context means that they will not cure your illness but will help you feel better and live longer), such as blood transfusions, palliative radiation or chemotherapy, and antibiotics, may be too expensive for hospice services to provide. A single blood transfusion can cost more than four days of hospice care, and a course of radiation can cost the same as two weeks of hospice services. As you can see, the math just doesn't add up.

The daily-payment method for hospice care frequently keeps people from enrolling in hospice sooner, which is a shame. When the hospice benefit was designed in 1982, this payment method made sense. Few palliative treatments were available for people nearing the end of life other than pain medicine, so the daily-payment model worked well. Over the years, however, the hospice payment hasn't kept up with advances in medical care. Recent changes by Medicare governing how hospices are paid (more in the first few weeks after enrollment and the last few weeks of life) may make it easier for people to receive these noncurative but helpful treatments. We'll have to see.

Besides wanting to continue disease-focused treatments that help them feel better and keep them alive, many patients wait to get hospice care until they have talked with their doctor about the possibility of getting additional disease-focused treatments. Often, these people are weak and have advanced illness. The message they get is, "Get stronger, and when you do, come see me so we can discuss giving you more disease-focused treatments." The trouble is that these patients are often at a stage where it's unrealistic to think that they'll get stronger. Don't wait. Enroll in hospice and reap the benefits now. If you do get stronger and want to take additional disease-focused treatments, you can be discharged from hospice.

> Virtually everyone who enrolls in hospice tells me, "I wish I had enrolled in hospice sooner." Don't let this happen to you. If you're not ready to commit to hospice because you're considering taking disease-focused treatments or you're hoping to get stronger, enroll in the meantime. If you are actively taking disease-focused treatments, ask your insurance company if it will pay for you to have hospice care along with those disease-focused treatments. Forward-thinking insurers are making this possible, and yours just might agree.

If you can't get your insurance company to agree to pay for hospice in addition to disease-focused treatments, ask your doctor or a social worker to intervene on your behalf. In California, Medicaid (Medi-Cal as it's called) allows seriously ill people to simultaneously get both palliative care or hospice care and disease-focused treatments. However, many Medicare recipients have to choose between hospice and curative treatments, though some Medicare Advantage programs provide both. If you have insurance coverage in addition to Medicare, one plan could pay for hospice while the other pays for disease-focused treatment. I hope Medicare will soon change its outdated rule.

If you reach a point where you're considering stopping disease-focused treatment or are worried that it's not helping, consider getting hospice care and seeing how it makes you feel. Remember, you can always change your mind and stop receiving hospice services, but you very well may decide not to.

If you receive hospice care, you're likely to feel stronger and better than you would have felt without it, and you'll be more likely to qualify for additional disease-directed treatment. Ironically, I find that most patients end up deciding not to take those disease-focused treatments and then lose out by not getting to spend as much time as they might have in hospice care. Those who do decide to take disease-directed treatments have the benefit of having had hospice services in the meantime.

WHAT HAPPENS WHEN YOU ENROLL IN HOSPICE?

When you're considering hospice care, a hospice nurse or social worker will meet with you to explain the service, assess your needs, and answer questions. This meeting can be in your home, the hospital, or a nursing home.

When you sign up for hospice services, a nurse will make a formal intake evaluation to understand how you're feeling physically, emotionally, psychologically, and spiritually. If you will remain at home, a nurse or social worker will come to your home to assess your needs. Often, equipment will have to be brought in and furniture rearranged. For example, changes may be required to accommodate a hospital bed, or your living room may have to become your bedroom to make access easier for you, your family, and hospice personnel.

The nurse, you, your family, the hospice team, and your doctor will develop a plan to address your needs. If needed, a social worker or chaplain will also see you. The nurse will talk to you about your values and goals and help you complete an advance health care directive and POLST form to clearly document your wishes.

The nurse will visit as often as needed to make sure you're comfortable. Initially, visits might be every day or three times a week. If your condition stabilizes and you're doing well, the nurse may only visit once a week or once a month. If you have new or worsening problems, including more pain, shortness of breath, or anxiety, or if your condition changes and you get weaker or near death, the nurse will generally visit and then come more frequently. In some hospice agencies, doctors may also make home visits.

If you have symptoms that need ongoing attention, a nurse can stay with you for eight-hour shifts. When your symptoms are so severe that you need a few days in a hospital or nursing home to get them under control, you don't need to disenroll from hospice. That care is part of hospice services. If your caregiver needs a break, someone can be sent to be with you for a few hours while your caregiver is away. That service is called respite care. Or you can be moved to a hospital, hospice facility, or nursing home for a few days of respite care.

If, in the middle of the night, you have a question, a concern, or an emergency, "call hospice, not 911." In fact, you can call hospice at any time because they provide around-the-clock telephone contact. If needed, they will send a nurse to see you at any time of day or night.

After hospice patients die, their families or caregivers can call hospice. Generally, someone will come to comfort survivors and help with arrangements such as calling the coroner and funeral home. In most cases, a hospice nurse or social worker will talk with you in advance about the funeral home you plan to use and can offer suggestions. While these conversations may seem a bit morbid, discussing important decisions beforehand helps dramatically when you're grieving after the death of your loved one.

VOLUNTEERS

Volunteers are an essential part of hospice care. They play a major role in the delivery of hospice services and the running of hospice organizations. Some hospice organizations have no paid employees and are staffed exclusively by volunteers. But most hospice organizations have paid staff and volunteers. The role of hospice volunteers is recognized by Medicare, which requires that volunteers provide at least 5 percent of patient-care hours in hospice. As a result, in 2014 about 430,000 people served as volunteers for hospices in the United States.

Most hospice volunteers provide direct service to patients and their families by helping to do whatever is necessary. Most commonly, they visit patients regularly, provide companionship, listen, and assist with household and personal chores. They also may provide help with childcare, run errands, arrange appointments, and provide transportation—whatever is needed.

Often, volunteers' greatest contribution is simply providing companionship: just being there with patients and their loved ones and letting them know that they are cared for and that they're not alone. If you enroll in hospice, chances are that a volunteer will help provide care and extend the reach and scope of the hospice team.

Most hospice volunteers undergo detailed personal background checks and health screenings. All volunteers are trained to know what to expect, what to do, what not to do, and who to contact in an emergency. Survivors of patients who received hospice care frequently want to volunteer, but most hospices require them to wait before serving.

BEREAVEMENT

Hospices provide grief and bereavement care for at least one year after a patient's death. They also keep in contact with and support deceased patients' loved ones. One of the toughest times for survivors is the anniversary of their loved one's death. While friends and even some family members may not be aware of those anniversaries, survivors are—acutely so. And so are hospices. They send cards to survivors, and knowing that someone is thinking of you on that sad and difficult day can be a great comfort. Many hospices also sponsor bereavement groups and provide support for anyone in the community who has experienced the death of a family member or friend or a similar loss.

RX

Hospice is a marvelous and invaluable service. It's readily available throughout the United States. Hospice is usually provided at home by a team of experts. Enrolling in hospice requires your doctor to state that you have a terminal illness and a prognosis of six months or less, but half of those who enroll receive care for only seventeen days. Longer hospice stays are associated with better quality of life near the end of life.

Don't be someone who says, "I wish I had started hospice sooner." If you're on the fence, try it. If you're continuing to pursue curative treatments or expensive palliative care treatments that are beyond what hospice can pay for, ask your health insurance company to pay for both. Many will. If your goal is to remain at home as much as possible while you deal with your illness, hospice care is a great way to reach that goal.

chapter fourteen

DIFFICULT TREATMENT DECISIONS AND DISCUSSIONS

THROUGHOUT YOUR ILLNESS, YOU'LL BE FACED WITH MA-
jor medical decisions. As you get closer to the end of life, the
stakes will get higher. When your illness progresses, the chances
that a treatment will make you better go down, and the odds that
it will make you weaker go up. For example, an operation you
might have sailed through when you were healthy can be devastating when you're weakened by cancer or heart failure.

As your condition deteriorates, surgery, chemotherapy, and
clinical trials can be tempting. I often hear patients say, "Why
not try it? What do I have to lose?" Actually, you can lose a
lot; you can have serious side effects and get little benefit. Too
many patients go for a last cycle of chemotherapy or have surgery from which they never recover. They land in the hospital
in worse condition than they were in prior to their chemo treat-

ment or surgery. Although the chances of success were slight, their hope for a miraculous cure took over and overruled common sense.

As you approach the end of life, be extremely careful what you agree to. Benefits may or may not come, but side effects will, and the risks and stakes are greater. Certain treatments may keep you alive, but in what condition? Instead of dying, you may live but be unable to function or enjoy what remains of your life. And some treatments may actually shorten your life. So as I've previously stressed, investigate all treatments, devices, and procedures before you agree to them.

Common treatments that we rarely question can have unfortunate consequences as you near the end. Antibiotics, special types of pacemakers called defibrillators, and surgery for bowel obstructions are three common examples:

Antibiotics: The risk of using antibiotics may seem slight since we've all taken them. However, when given near the end of life, it's not clear whether they help you live better or just prolong the dying process. If you're thinking about starting antibiotics because an infection is causing discomfort, consider treating the discomfort directly—for example, with pain medicine. If you consider antibiotics to treat the fever associated with infection, better and faster alternatives exist to treat a fever directly. Antibiotics are not without risk. They can cause diarrhea and rashes and may require you to get another IV.

Don't start antibiotics because you can or as a knee-jerk reaction to the possibility of infection. Ask the hard but important questions about what the antibiotic will do to help you or your loved one. And also ask about the risks.

> neumonia was once called "the old man's friend" be-
> cause it afflicted those who were nearing the end of
> life and allowed them to die relatively quickly. Now antibi-
> otics can be effective against pneumonia and prolong life,
> but at what price?

Pacemakers: Heart failure patients often receive pacemakers that include implantable cardioverter defibrillators (ICDs). Pacemakers keep your heart rhythm steady when the electrical system isn't functioning properly. The ICD function shocks your heart if it starts beating abnormally fast, in hopes of getting it to resume beating normally. An ICD only provides a shock if your heart starts to beat in a dangerous manner that could cause death in a matter of minutes or seconds. While ICDs prevent sudden death from abnormal heart rhythms, at the end of life they may prevent you from having exactly what you hope for—a sudden, quick, and painless death, preferably in your sleep. Many patients think that their ICD is keeping them alive, but it's actually just preventing sudden death. On the other hand, the pacemaker function often helps to keep you comfortable—for example, by preventing an abnormally slow heart rate. Since these devices are very sophisticated, it's possible to turn off the ICD feature and leave the pacemaker working.

Surgery for bowel obstruction: Cancer patients, especially those who have cancer in the abdomen such as colon cancer, pancreatic cancer, or ovarian cancer, commonly get bowel obstructions. Their bowels get blocked, and food and water can't get through. They experience cramping, pain, nausea, and vomiting. Bowel obstructions can come and go or come and stay. They can vary in severity: sometimes you can eat and drink a little, but other times you can't eat or drink at all.

It is tempting to want to treat a bowel obstruction due to cancer with surgery. We imagine that our bowels are like the pipes in our house. If a blockage occurs in a pipe, we can just cut out the blocked section and reconnect the two pieces. However, our bodies don't work that way. Surgery for bowel obstructions during late-stage cancer rarely helps. It is a classic example of wanting to make something better but making it worse than if you had left it alone. In advanced cancer, the best approach is to use medicines to relieve pain and help the bowel rest.

CULTURE AND TRADITIONS

Serious illness doesn't discriminate; it strikes patients of all ethnic and cultural backgrounds. Members of particular groups frequently have traditions that govern how they deal with serious illness, dying, and death.

In today's Western cultures, the wishes of seriously ill people are paramount. Our laws and institutions are geared toward seeing that their directives are carried out. In other cultures, decisions are based on what's best for the family, and the individual's interests are less important. The patient's family, not the patient, is expected to make the important decisions, including treatment and end-of-life decisions.

If you want your family to make those decisions, make your wishes clear. Put them in writing. Make sure that they're in your medical record. Tell your family, friends, and medical providers that you authorize your family to make all the necessary decisions regarding your treatment and end-of-life care.

When it comes to cultural differences, my major concern is that assumptions will be made that don't reflect patients' wishes.

I was treating Mae, a Chinese-American patient in the ICU, when it became clear that she had only a matter of days left. I asked her nurse, who was also Chinese-American, if she knew whether anyone had asked about Mae's spiritual preferences. Did she want to see a spiritual leader or have particular customs followed? "Oh, no," the nurse replied, "we Chinese aren't religious." Her answer surprised me. It was not what I had experienced. So I asked Mae's family, learned that they were Catholic, and was told that both Mae and her family wanted her to receive the Sacrament of the Sick, which we soon arranged.

You can't assume that you know about someone because you know their ethnicity, country of origin, religion, or primary language. You certainly don't know their preferences for something as personal as medical care and spiritual needs at the end of life.

Although cultural traditions play a role in making treatment decisions, that role is not absolute. For example, in some cultures the tradition is to withhold unfavorable information from patients. In those cultures, physicians don't discuss diagnosis and prognosis directly with the patient. And yet, cultures are not homogeneous. Opinions diverge even in the most traditional communities. They are never 100 percent one way or the other. Ultimately, treatment and end-of-life decisions are personal and vary with each case.

I tell my students to be curious. To ask respectful questions like, "What do I need to know about your culture or religion to make sure I take good care of you?" Share these traditions and practices with your doctors and nurses. If the person who is ill in your family is potentially more traditional than you are, you can ask them the same question: "Grandma, what are the traditions in our family that are important when taking care of people who are sick?" This question about traditions is another opportunity for the person who is sick to find meaning, purpose, legacy, and dignity by sharing family and cultural traditions.

On the other hand, I sometimes find that people don't want straight talk. Some people prefer to be a bit in the dark, to live with some denial. That's OK too. The point is that you can never know what someone will say. That goes for me as a doctor and for family members. The goal is not to assume what someone wants but to ask.

At eighty-four, Mr. Wong was admitted to the hospital with right-sided abdominal pain. An ultrasound revealed a mass in his gallbladder that looked like cancer. His family told us not to tell him what we found because he wouldn't be able to take such bad news. They said that, in their tradition, the family would make all medical decisions for him.

One morning, when Mr. Wong was feeling better, I visited him. He was in bed, and a Mandarin interpreter was with his family in the room. I wanted to respect the family's wish, but I also wanted to respect Mr. Wong. So I said, "Mr. Wong, I have information about what's going on. Some people want me to tell them everything, while others prefer that I only speak to their families. How do you feel?"

Mr. Wong thought for a moment and then spoke in Mandarin, which the interpreter translated. "You know, Doctor, everyone has to die someday." I was stunned. I hadn't said anything about dying. I regrouped and said that yes, he was right, but what I wanted to know was how he wanted me to handle new information about his condition and whether he wanted me to tell him or his family. "Oh, doctor," he replied, "you will tell me everything. And by the way, it's OK if you also want to tell my family."

Mr. Wong went on to tell us that he felt better and wanted to go home. He declined a biopsy that his family had been ready to consent to. Mr. Wong's family thought they were protecting him, but they had complicated the situation and made it more difficult. They nearly exposed him to a biopsy that he didn't want.

> The federal government, along with every state in the United States, has laws that mandate that health care providers make interpreters available for any person who doesn't speak English [14.1]. These laws are so important because they support better patient-doctor and patient-nurse communication, which is the backbone of good medical care.

FAMILY WORRIES

People from all cultures and walks of life worry about how their loved one will respond to hearing bad news. I'm often told, "Don't tell my mother that she has cancer," or "Don't tell my dad that he's dying." They're afraid that this information will be too devastating for their loved one, that the news will literally kill them. They ignore the fact that the patient, a brilliant college professor, for example, has been coming to a building called "the Cancer Center" for months.

By and large, patients know when they're very sick and approaching the end of life. They know how they feel; they know that they're getting weaker. Patients hear the hushed tones outside their rooms. Everyone treats them too nicely. Family and friends cry when talking to them, and visitors suddenly arrive from the four corners of the earth. Your loved ones don't cross borders for pneumonia, but they cross the ocean if you are dying from lung cancer.

I realize that when I ask patients, like Mr. Wong, how I should handle information about their illness, they will conclude that the news is bad. If the news were good, they reason, I wouldn't ask. And they are right. Still, the question enables patients who don't want information to decline hearing it, and ultimately, what we want is to respect each person's feelings and beliefs.

When Mrs. Parvaz was hospitalized for advanced cancer, her family told me not to tell her that she was dying. They didn't think she could handle it. I told her husband and daughters that I would ask her what she wanted to know and would respect her wishes. They agreed but didn't want to be present during that conversation for fear that they would start crying and telegraph the bad news.

When I asked Mrs. Parvaz, she said that she wanted to know everything and that she wanted it straight with no mincing of words. I explained that the cancer was very advanced and that she had only days or weeks to live. Mrs. Parvaz was sad but not surprised given how weak she felt. She asked me to send her family members in one by one because she had things to tell each of them, and now was the time.

Our conversation motivated Mrs. Parvaz to speak freely to her loved ones, to express her feelings, and to give them important information that she had been thinking about but couldn't find the right time to share. Mrs. Parvaz and her family were grateful for the opportunity to talk so intimately—an opportunity they otherwise might have missed.

Treat your loved ones with the same respect you would want for yourself. When I ask families what they would do if the tables were turned, they invariably say that they would want to hear the information directly. In addition, recognize that when you avoid talking about what's going on, you isolate the person who is sick. Ask them if they want to receive news about their condition from their medical team, or if they would prefer having their doctors and nurses tell their family. You may be surprised by their answers.

TALKING WITH CHILDREN

When a parent is dying, it turns a child's world upside down. Everything the child needs—love, consistency, support, routine, attention, access to parents—is torn apart. Dying parents may be too weak or tired to care for or even spend time with their children; they may be immobile, be incapacitated, look different, and need their own support. Children, especially young children, fear separation from their parents, and having their routines disrupted can make them feel uncertain, frightened, and insecure. They need structure, reassurance, and support.

Although we desperately want to protect children from the pain of loss, we can't shield them from a parent's death. Trying to can backfire and make matters worse. Open and honest communication targeted to the child's age and ability to understand can minimize the long- and short-term emotional impact of a parent's death. Not talking with them about it doesn't mean that they won't know what is happening. Children are perceptive. They can sense what's going on, and if they're not told, they may become distrustful, angry, resentful, and withdrawn. You can even include children in conversations with doctors and nurses so they hear the information directly, but you'll probably have to answer their questions afterward.

A child's age matters in how they respond to the loss of a parent because children of different ages experience the world differently. However, some common messages are appropriate for all:

> Mommy's/Daddy's condition has changed, and she/he is now much sicker.
> This is what is really happening . . .
> You are not the cause of this illness. Illness just happens.
> Someone will take care of you no matter what happens, and that someone is ___.

After their parent dies, tell children clearly but simply and compassionately. "I'm so sorry, but Mommy has died." Avoid euphemisms like "Mommy went to God" or "Daddy has passed on." Be prepared for any reaction, from wailing to calm, as the child figures it out. Stay attentive and be patient and available.

Issues involved with telling children vary with their ages and developmental stages. Keep in mind that some children are more (or less) advanced and that in the face of stress, they may regress and act younger than their age.

Infants and toddlers up to age two need routine, especially around bedtimes and mealtimes, as well as a small group of attentive, predictable, consistent, and loving caregivers.

Preschoolers aged three to five years don't understand that death is permanent. They are also very concrete thinkers. In explaining death, it is important to describe what happens: "Mommy's body isn't working, and she can't move or breathe anymore." Telling preschoolers that "Mommy went to sleep" may make them fear going to bed and not waking up. Expect these children to ask the same questions over and over again.

School-aged children aged six to twelve years are starting to understand the permanence of death and may focus on the physical aspects of it. They also may ask questions that make you uncomfortable, such as "How do you eat when you die?" Since these children may not understand spiritual or metaphysical explanations, saying "Daddy's soul is going to heaven" may have no meaning to them. If you explain how the body is dealt with in your tradition—for example, by burial or cremation—the child may ask if Mommy will get cold underground or if cremation hurts. At this age, children spend much of their day at school, so it's important to notify their teachers and administrators about the situation.

Adolescents aged thirteen years and up have a full and adult level of understanding of what death means. They are struggling with their own individuation and separation from their parents, so permanent separation as a result of death is especially difficult. They may move from thinking about the spiritual implications of death to concrete concerns about what their parent's death will mean to them. Adolescents can be self-absorbed, which should not be misinterpreted as being unfeeling, indifferent, or insensitive. Older and more mature adolescents may want and need the same type of information that adults want.

As for visiting or spending time with the dying parent, let the children lead. Asking the children directly if they would like to visit will let you know their wishes and indicate their readiness. If they want to visit, let them. If not, don't force them. Prepare them for hospital visits by explaining what they're going to see: IVs, intubation, or little or no response. Showing them photographs before the visit can help them decide whether to visit and prepare them for what they'll see. Assign a companion for all visits and create a code so children can signal when they want to leave.

Regardless of whether the children want to visit, they may want to make a card, draw a picture, write a letter, or make a video for their parent. Children may not vocalize their feelings and instead express emotions through art and play. Providing these opportunities can be very helpful.

Parents: Think about the legacy you want to leave your children. Write letters to them that can be read after you're gone and at milestones such as graduations, confirmations, bar mitzvahs, weddings, and special occasions. Leave them personalized gifts and special mementos and record an audio or video message. I discuss legacy in more detail in chapter 10.

RX

With serious illness, there is typically a series of decisions to be made about treatments. Cultural issues are important so don't assume that you know what your loved one wants or what decisions they will make. There is no one right answer, though I find that talking is always better than silence.

chapter fifteen

THE END: WHAT IS IT LIKE?

WE'RE ALL CONCERNED WITH HOW THE FINAL CHAPTER OF our lives will end. When we think about death, we're filled with questions and fears. Will it be painful, distressing, or hard? How will we know? When will it happen? What will we feel? What comes next?

I can't say that I have answers. If it were up to me, we would live with all our faculties intact until we were very old and then go quietly in our sleep. But, alas, life generally doesn't work that way. Serious illness is the norm.

Most of the time, the end of life is peaceful. Most seriously ill people die quietly, without drama. Rarely do they have startling awakenings, lucid moments, or periods of clarity where they make profound final statements, grand gestures, or significant reconciliations. Unlike those dramatic movie death scenes, most people go without fanfare; they peacefully slip away.

Mrs. Caldwell was in her late eighties and had advanced dementia. She was admitted to the hospital because she had pneumonia and difficulty breathing. Her son, reflecting his mother's wishes, decided against antibiotics and told us that his mother would want us to focus only on her comfort. When I entered her hospital room, her son, who had been steadily by her side for the past three days, was sitting on a couch a few feet from her bed, reading the *San Francisco Chronicle*. "Good morning," I said. "How's she doing?" "She had a quiet night," he replied.

As I approached Mrs. Caldwell, I noticed that she wasn't breathing, which isn't uncommon. Patients at the end of life often have long pauses in their breathing, but in this case, Mrs. Caldwell hadn't just paused, she had died. She was so peaceful that her son hadn't realized that her breathing had stopped and she had died.

SIGNS THAT THE END IS NEAR

How will you know that you're nearing the end of life? Certain signs indicate that we're getting closer to death—the most important of which is how much we can still do for ourselves. As illness progresses, our bodies get weaker. We tend to spend more time resting in bed or a chair, we have a harder time getting around, and progressively, we're less able to care for ourselves. We need help bathing, dressing, getting out of bed, and going to the bathroom. For example, when patients who have metastatic cancer spend half their waking hours in a bed or a chair, their prognosis is about two to three months.

Some people get weaker gradually; it can take months or years. Patients who are healthier when they're diagnosed often maintain their physical prowess until late in their illnesses and then decline rapidly—frequently in a matter of weeks. It's both the gift and the curse of having a young and otherwise healthy body when you're found to have a serious illness.

During the last weeks of life, our bodies start to shut down. We lose weight, eat less, stay in bed more, sleep longer, and even have bowel movements less frequently. Many of us become more inwardly focused and want calm, quiet, and fewer visitors. We can feel as if our world has shrunk, and we have no interest in going out, even out of our bedroom.

Patients' family and friends find these changes chilling and hard to accept. Watching a loved one get weaker and pull away is frightening. Families beg their loved ones to hang on and fight. They become cheerleaders and try to forestall their loved ones' decline by providing food, stimulus, and encouragement. They bring in people to entertain them, energize them, and lift their spirits. It's important to recognize and respect these changes and to match your energy to the patient's energy.

NUTRITION AND HYDRATION

When they near the end of life, people stop eating. Family and friends often tell me that their loved ones are dying because they're not eating and that they would get stronger if they ate more. The fact is, *people stop eating because they're dying*, not the other way around. In just about every serious illness, people stop eating as they near the end of life. Unfortunately, eating more doesn't make terminally ill patients stronger or help them live longer.

In the early stages of serious illness, good nutrition is essential. It gives patients the strength to deal with their illness and their treatments. However, at the end of life, most people are not hungry or thirsty, and those who are tend to need very little food or water to relieve their hunger or thirst. When we stop eating near the end of life, our bodies break down fat for energy, and that process generates water that our bodies can use. It's remarkable how little some patients drink at the end of life and still produce clear urine.

I'm often told, "But Dr. Pantilat, she is going to starve to death." This fear is so common that I usually address it before I hear it from patients' loved ones. The thought that someone you love is starving is horrifying and hard to take. Our instinct is to feed them. I try to explain as gently and compassionately as possible to families and friends that their loved ones aren't starving—they're dying from their illness. Losing weight, eating less, or not eating at all is part of the dying process.

When patients stop eating or eat very little, we're often asked about giving them artificial nutrition and fluids. Patients and families frequently want us to supplement the patients' nutrition through feeding tubes or IVs. I tell them that I wish artificial nutrition were the answer; I wish that a few good meals or putting nutrition directly into their bloodstreams through IVs would get them back on their feet. However, it's not that easy.

When patients have diseases such as cancer or lung and heart disease, the body produces hormones that cause their bodies to waste away and not use the nutrition they're given. It's as if the body is trying to deny the illness energy, but in the process, it's also denying itself. The belief that nutrition will help is so strong and the fact that it won't help so counterintuitive, that it's been extensively studied. However, study after study has confirmed that artificial nutrition via feeding tubes or IVs doesn't help those who are dying get stronger, be more awake, or live longer [15.1].

Plus, giving patients artificial nutrition has downsides. Feeding tubes are uncomfortable. They're worth the discomfort if they help, but they don't help at the end of life. They also can cause complications including pneumonia and diarrhea. Nutrition by IV is worse and can increase your chances of getting blood infections.

It's not that artificial nutrition is never helpful. For people undergoing bone marrow transplants and those with sudden, critical illness in the ICU, recovery often hinges on receiving artificial nutrition. However, near the end of life, these treatments no longer work, they can be dangerous, and they can cause more harm than good. This fact is one of the most counterintuitive and difficult for patients and their families to accept, but it's true.

The best approach is to offer your loved ones whatever they want to eat and drink. Accept the fact that they may eat and drink very little. Find other ways to show your love and concern, like holding their hand, reading to them, and telling them you love them.

THE VERY END

One hundred years ago, most people died at home and were with someone as they died. Today, so many people die in hospitals and families are so scattered that it's less common for you to witness a death at home. Being with someone who is dying is a profound and intimate experience. You might find it spiritual. As a physician, I've been at the bedside of many people at the moment of death. Most were hospitalized, but a few were at home. Witnessing death never fails to move me.

We often worry that death will be out of control or frightening. Usually, it's peaceful. In the final hours and days, death from serious illness doesn't follow a constant, uniform path, but it has common signs. Knowing those signs, understanding how the end may unfold, is important in easing stress and worry. Be observant and ask questions about what you notice that seems unusual. What is normal at the end of life differs from what is normal otherwise. Knowing what to expect as your loved one is dying is associated with an easier time in bereavement and a lower risk of complicated grief.

In life's final hours and days, people go through changes as their bodies shut down. I will explain the most common changes that occur so that if you observe them you will understand what they mean, and what, if anything, to do about them:

Level of consciousness: In the final hours or days, it's common to become less alert. In fact, it's rare for those near death to be awake and conversant. Near the end, many drift in and out of consciousness, which is called delirium. Most often, delirium isn't distressing. Those who are more awake may try to speak but be incoherent. They can have visions or hear voices, which are often pleasant. My grandfather saw his mother in a white gown in his final days. He hadn't seen her since he left Poland sixty years earlier. Most delirium doesn't need treatment.

Occasionally, people will have agitated delirium. They'll drift in and out of consciousness, and when awake, they may be restless and agitated. They may thrash around, try to get out of bed, and cry out. Agitated delirium can be frightening and distressing to watch. It has many causes: pain, bladder infection, constipation, and the side effects of medications. When those who are not at the end of life have agitated delirium, we try to uncover the cause and treat it. At the very end of life, we treat the agitation directly and concentrate on making sure that delirious patients don't get hurt.

If you observe agitated delirium, immediately get help, because medications such as haloperidol are effective when promptly given. Speak to your loved one in a calm voice, touch him or her gently, and try to help him or her calm down. If the individual is enrolled in hospice, call the hospice. They may have left medicine at your home in an emergency kit and can instruct you to use it. If your loved one is not enrolled in hospice, call your doctor. If your loved one is in the hospital or a nursing home, call the nurse.

> ### CAN SHE HEAR ME?
>
> When your loved one is unconscious or barely conscious, it can be impossible to communicate with him or her. Family members often ask me, "Can she hear me?" I answer that we have no way to know for sure. I've noticed that patients who are dying seem to respond differently to familiar voices than they do to mine. They seem to get calmer when they hear a loved one's voice. We also know that hearing is one of the last senses to go.
>
> I always tell people, "Say what you want to say and whatever is in your heart." As I suggested in chapter 10, think about saying, "Forgive me. I forgive you. Thank you. I love you. Good-bye." It is likely that your loved one has a sense that you're there. If you can't be at your loved one's bedside, speak to him or her by phone. Ask an attendant to put the receiver up to his or her ear. Simply saying your piece has great power, regardless of whether you get a response.

Breathing patterns: When people are dying, their breathing patterns change. They may breathe very slowly, only taking three or four breaths a minute. Or they may take a few breaths and then pause for thirty, forty, or fifty seconds before they take another breath. If you're at their bedside, it can be distressing and you may think after every breath that it was their last one. Then, just when you think they won't take another breath, they suddenly do.

Another common pattern is what doctors and nurses call Cheyne-Stokes respiration: the breathing oscillates from very fast to slow, then to a pause, and then fast again. This pattern results from the brain being less sensitive to the stimulus to breathe, so breathing falls behind, but then catches up, overdoes it, and then falls behind again. Cheyne-Stokes respiration is normal at the end of life.

Some people will take very deep, consecutive breaths one after another. This pattern is less common but still normal. You may also notice that your loved one may alternate between patterns.

As people die, they may also take extremely shallow breaths and exhale very little air. Typically, these are final breaths—when the body is too weak to breathe fully. When you see such shallow breaths, the end is at hand: usually hours or minutes away.

None of these breathing patterns requires treatment. The only pattern that usually needs to be treated is very fast breathing. Although doctors differ on how fast is too fast, I consider anything more than thirty breaths a minute too fast. I think that if a breathing pattern would be uncomfortable if the patient were awake, and breathing thirty times a minute lying in bed would be uncomfortable, then it should be treated. As I wrote in chapter 6, oxygen is helpful only if the patient's oxygen level is low. The trouble is that at the end of life, oxygen levels are low and will get lower. So oxygen is not usually the right answer. However, if it was already being used, it may be fine to continue it.

I often stop oxygen when patients are actively dying because it's doing them little good, and stopping it usually has no negative effect. Supplemental oxygen can prolong the dying process, and the tubes and masks prevent loved ones from caressing and kissing the patient's face. Fresh air through an open window or a fan can be helpful. And opioids, as I describe in chapter 6, are the most effective medication for shortness of breath.

Rattle: People who are dying are too weak to swallow their saliva and phlegm or to cough it up, so it pools in the back of their throats. As they breathe, air travels over this collection of fluid and makes a rattling sound, which can get quite loud and be distressing to hear, although it doesn't seem to be uncomfortable for the patient. Though many medications have been tested to reduce this noise, none have worked. Resist the impulse to try suctioning, as it's uncomfortable. The best approach is to turn the patient to one side. It will then take a while for the fluid to re-accumulate, but in the meantime the rattle will probably get softer or disappear.

Hands and feet: Just before death, hands and feet can become mottled, turn blue or purplish, and get cold. These changes are also signs that the body is shutting down and the patient's circulation is poor. I've also observed swelling in the back of the hand, even in people without IVs. I can't explain why it occurs, but I've seen it enough to find it a useful sign of imminent death. Usually, these changes in the hands and feet mean that death will occur that day.

Lucid periods before death are rare but can occur. I've witnessed it many times. At first, it can be a bit jarring. You expect your loved one to continue to fade, and suddenly he or she awakens. Some see it as a sign of improvement or recovery, but in my experience these episodes are short lived. If your loved one has a lucid interval, enjoy it. Use it to express your love and gratitude.

IT COULD HAPPEN SUDDENLY

When I care for patients at the end of their lives, I let their family and friends know what to expect, and I list the signs that indicate that they're nearing death. Still, it's not an exact science. Sick people can and do die suddenly, without warning—especially those with heart failure, for whom sudden death is common.

Since sudden deaths are frequent among those nearing the end of life, I tell families that want to be sure to be with their loved ones when they die not to leave their bedsides. It's not uncommon for patients to seem stable and for family members, after being there for days, to step out for a break only to return ten minutes later to find that their loved one has died. I've seen this so often that I developed a theory: I think dying patients have a sense of their impending deaths. So they choose the moment when they're alone to die. It's as though it's too hard to leave their loved ones or to subject them to seeing them die. I've seen this too many times to think it's just coincidence, although I have no scientific explanation for this theory. If it is very important for you to have someone with your loved one at the moment of death, make arrangements to have someone there all the time.

If your loved one dies when you've stepped away, don't feel guilty. I've heard many family members say, "I abandoned my mother when she died." Some people carry this guilt for the rest of their lives. Let it go. Consider that it happened that way on purpose. The moment of death can be intimate and profound, but it's not the most important moment. The most important moments occur over the course of a lifetime; they're the moments when you share life.

Knowing that the unexpected can and will happen is vital, because it can be a shock when your loved one dies—even though you knew it was coming and expected it. Being prepared won't take away your sadness and grief, but it can ease the shock.

We all try to make sense of what has happened and explain it. Sometimes our explanations are misplaced and create stress and compound our grief. Focus on the good times you spent with your loved one, the special experiences, and the many times you shared treasured moments. If your loved one dies alone, consider that he or she may have wanted it that way.

> ### SHOULD I VISIT NOW?
>
> Family members often contact me to ask on behalf of people who live far away whether they should visit. They're really asking whether this is the end, because they feel it's important for them to be with their loved one and their family at the time of death.
>
> If you're thinking of visiting a loved one who is seriously ill, *do it now*. Don't wait until the end. Near the end of life, your loved one may not be conscious or able to communicate. Visit early and often while you can still have meaningful visits. If your loved one rallies, you can always visit again. And if he or she dies before you had the chance to return, you'll have had a meaningful visit. Whenever you leave, say good-bye, thank you, and I love you.

WHAT YOU CAN DO

Managing your loved one's care at home can seem overwhelming. Get help, because it's a full-time, around-the-clock job. If your loved one wants to die at home, it can be challenging for you but doable. Enroll your loved one in hospice or home palliative care. Speak with the doctors and nurses from those services and get their advice. Recruit family and friends and hire help. Review chapters 6 and 8 on managing pain and caregiving.

Try to remember what your loved one would like. What would make him or her happy? My rule is that whatever patients liked when they were well, they will probably like when they're dying. Conversely, what they previously disliked, they usually won't like now. That goes for music, poetry, massage, singing, and holding hands.

Try to make your loved one comfortable. If he or she is unconscious, moisten his or her lips with a towel and apply balm for chapped lips. Tell stories of your life together. I find storytelling especially helpful. It reminds you of happier times and moments you shared and is a great way to let others, particularly those who are younger, learn about the person who is dying. Also express your love, gratitude, and appreciation. Tell them how proud you've always been of them. Assure them that you'll take care of whatever is most important to them.

> When you visit patients, match your energy to the energy in the room. If the room is peaceful, don't come bounding in bright and bubbly, but also don't brood or be grim and gloomy. If the atmosphere is quiet, speak softly and sparingly. Understand that the energy in the room reflects the patient's feelings and state of mind and indicates how you should act.

All families have their own quirks, unique relationships, and levels of dysfunction. Nothing about serious illness or the end of life changes that. When a loved one is dying, it would be great if we all could get along, stop bickering, rally, and find our best selves. Unfortunately, when we're at the bedside of a dying loved one, the stress can heighten pre-existing family dysfunction. Tempers can flare. Emotions can run high.

If someone is hurtful, attribute it to stress. Let it pass, give them room, and focus on your loved one. Think twice or even three times before you say anything that you might regret. Going forward, these people will still be your family. So take a break from old grudges, resentments, and hurt feelings to come together.

Opioids at the end of life: Most patients near the end of life take medication. Often, they're given opioids for their pain or shortness of breath, which you may have to administer. To keep your loved one comfortable, you may need to give opioids every couple of hours. When you give opioids this frequently, the patient will die within two hours of the last dose or quite possibly, sooner. Often, the person who gave that last dose thinks that she contributed to the death of her loved one, or worse, thinks that she outright killed him.

If you find yourself in this situation, don't blame yourself for contributing to your loved one's death. When a patient is dying from serious illness, he or she may have symptoms that must be relieved. The symptoms often require opioids, and sometimes large doses. Large opioid doses can hasten death and even cause it, but giving opioids to a dying person doesn't mean that you killed them. Those who are dying receive opioids because they're in pain; they don't die from being given opioids.

Treat your loved one's symptoms and don't hold back. No dying person should suffer needlessly. If your loved one dies soon after his or her last opioid dose, know that you did your best to provide good care, the timing was coincidental, and the opioids were not the cause of death.

SETTINGS

Decide where you want to be at the end of your life. A quarter of Americans die in hospitals, and nearly one-third spend time in an ICU in the last month of life. Another 28 percent die in nursing homes, and one-third die at home.

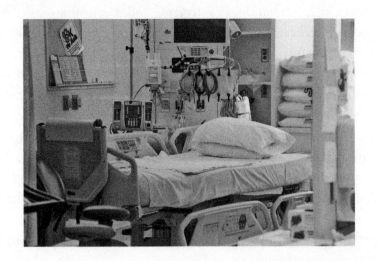

When I talk to groups, I ask my audiences to imagine the end of their lives. Specifically, I ask them to picture where they are, who they're with, and what it looks like. Then I show them a picture of an ICU and ask, "How many of you want this?" No one ever raises their hand.

While most people want to die at home, it's not a priority for others. They may feel more secure in the hospital or think they'll get better care. The challenge is that hospitals are not set up to be peaceful and quiet, and they're not ideal venues for intimate visits. Hospitals are noisy; they're hubs of constant activity. Machines buzz, intercoms go off, voices carry, and people scurry in and out endlessly. And ICUs are even more intense.

Finding dignity and comfort in an ICU is difficult. ICU patients are human pincushions. They have IVs inserted in their chests, necks, wrists, and feet. Compression stockings strangle their legs, and tubes plunge down their throats. Monitors are connected to their chest and fingers, and they're constantly being poked and prodded for injections, blood draws, and other tests. The noise is loud and steady, and privacy is a challenge.

Although intubation, IVs, oxygen, and medications are often lifesaving and can seem harmless once they are in place, they're hard on patients. After a while, even oxygen therapy can be irritating. Dealing with all the discomfort saps energy. One of my colleagues, Dr. Dan Burkhardt, an ICU specialist at UCSF, compares being in the ICU to getting a filling done at the dentist's office. Even though our mouths are numb and we don't feel pain, hearing the drill and having all that hardware in our mouths is far from comfortable. Now, imagine that experience, but a hundred times more invasive, involving your entire body 24/7. If you have a chance of recovery, it's worth it. But, if despite all the treatments you're still dying, then the ICU interventions will simply add to your suffering.

In the ICU, dying patients look exhausted. Many never wake up or get to interact with their loved ones because they're so sedated or lack the strength. They seem miserable and look ghostly and nothing like themselves. If the patient's goal is to die peacefully, we can disconnect the machines and provide medicines that promote comfort and ease pain. Often, conversations about this shift in care focus on what we'll stop or withdraw—the intubation, the dialysis, the antibiotics. It is important to emphasize that while the type of care we provide may shift, the *caring* will continue.

Any tube, including a breathing tube inserted into the throat, can be removed. Any monitor or machine can be disconnected. When they are, patients look much more peaceful, calm, and like themselves. Finally, they don't have to resist all the invasions and they can relax. Then, when patients are stable, we can move them from the ICU to more private and peaceful settings.

At UCSF and many other hospitals, these more peaceful settings are rooms that have been specially designed for patients who are dying and are too sick to leave the hospital. We call ours Comfort Care suites. They're bigger and more homelike in order to accommodate more family members and friends. Our Comfort Care suites are located at the end of the hall, so they are quieter, and they are not connected to the intercom. Medical equipment is kept in a cabinet where it's out of sight but available if needed. We also have foldout couches for loved ones who wish to spend the night, and we provide snacks for families.

Our Comfort Care suites are nice, but by no means as nice as a real home. However, they're oases away from the constant noise—retreats where patients and their families can have greater intimacy, dignity, and comfort. These special rooms can be havens for grieving families and friends.

> If, at the end of life, you or your loved one is hospitalized, ask for a palliative care consultation and ask that you be moved to a palliative care suite or similar type of room.

To sum up: hospitals, and especially ICUs, are not ideal places to die. They're institutional and noisy, they lack privacy, and they can overly medicalize a natural process. On the other hand, hospitals can provide comfort and dignity for patients who have symptoms that cannot be controlled at home. In my experience, excellent end-of-life care can be provided in any setting, but you have to get the right help. That help can come from hospice or palliative care teams or your personal doctor.

AID IN DYING

In recent years, "aid in dying" has been the subject of a great deal of passionate debate. Much of the recent discussion was generated by the widely reported case of Brittany Maynard, a twenty-nine-year-old Californian who moved to Oregon in order to end her life via aid in dying. Ms. Maynard had brain cancer and decided to end her life at the time of her choosing, which was not legally permissible in California at the time. Her case helped lead to the passage of California's End of Life Option Act, which took effect in June 2016.

Aid in dying is also called assisted suicide, physician-assisted suicide, physician aid in dying, compassionate death, and death with dignity. It occurs when a terminally ill patient requests, receives, and then takes a prescription from a doctor for medication that will end his or her life. Aid in dying doesn't allow physicians to give you a shot to end your life, which is illegal throughout the United States. It doesn't permit others to administer medicines to you to end your life. That's also illegal nationwide. In the states where aid in dying is legal, it is not considered suicide and is not permitted for those who are actively suicidal.

Sharp divisions exist over whether states should give their terminally ill citizens the legal right to receive and take a lethal prescription from a doctor to end their lives. Traditionally, our culture and religious faiths have favored natural death and prohibited our assisting in the death of others. In most states, aid in dying is illegal. Opponents of it believe that doctors have a moral duty to care for patients, which doesn't include helping them die, and that legalizing aid in dying would open a Pandora's box of troubling medical, legal, and moral questions.

> Those in favor of aid in dying say that it's a matter of dignity—having the ability to control your own life and death.
> Those opposed to it say that prohibiting aid in dying is a matter of dignity—protecting the dignity of human life.

Both sides argue their positions fervently.

Many seriously ill people think about taking their lives, but very few actually do. The will to live is extremely powerful, even for those who are seriously ill and in agonizing pain. For most people, the idea of shortening their lives is unfathomable. No one values a day more than those who have only a few days to live.

For those who are dying and want aid in dying, it's a matter of dignity and control. They seek the legal right to put their fate in their own hands, to avoid prolonged suffering, for themselves and their families, while their bodies waste away. They wish to choose the time and manner of their death and to have doctors assist them.

In the states where aid in dying is legal, it's rare. Those who consider it usually feel that control of their lives is of paramount importance. You might think that people opt for aid in dying because they have unrelenting pain, but that's rarely the reason they choose it. In Oregon, where it's been legal the longest, since 1997, many more people discuss aid in dying with their doctors than get prescriptions for medications. Few of those who get prescriptions actually fill them. Of those who fill their prescriptions, one-third never take them. For a detailed report on Oregon's Death with Dignity Act, visit www.healthoregon .org/dwd.

Just getting or filling the prescription can give seriously ill people emotional relief. Knowing that they can control their destiny and stop their suffering can be a comfort to them. They see their prescription as a last resort, a way out when their quality of life becomes unbearable.

As a doctor, I want to know if my patient is considering aid in dying, and I want to talk to him or her about it. When a patient raises the issue with me, I see it as a call for help and an expression of worry about the future that deserves immediate attention. I always say, "I'm glad you brought this up. Why are you thinking about this today?" I want to understand the concerns behind the request. Often, I can provide reassurance about their fears and worries and make plans for the future, including a referral to palliative care and hospice.

If you're considering aid in dying, you should also talk about it with your loved ones. Consider the impact your decision will have on your survivors, those who care for you, and your legacy. Of course it's your decision, but it's one that could have a big impact on your family and friends. You may find that your loved ones fully support your decision.

> Contemplating aid in dying is an expression of concern; it also can be a cry for help. It comes from worries about having intractable pain, feeling out of control, and being a burden. Those who seriously consider aid in dying think of it as a way to allay their fears and gain control.
>
> If you're thinking about aid in dying or ending your life, speak with your doctor as soon as possible. Tell your doctor about your fears and concerns. Get your doctor's perspective and advice, learn about your options, and get in-depth information on what you can do.

REQUIREMENTS

Aid in dying is legal in Oregon, Washington, Vermont, Colorado, and California. Physicians in those jurisdictions cannot be prosecuted for prescribing lethal medications for terminally ill patients if they follow detailed procedures outlined by law. The Supreme Court of Montana has also protected doctors in the state who participate in aid in dying. Aid in dying is statutorily prohibited in thirty-eight states, and in three states it violates the common law.

The laws in states permitting aid in dying are similar, but they vary to some degree. If your state permits aid in dying and you're considering it, check the requirements. In general, the legal requirements include the following:

You must be:

> At least eighteen years old.
> A state resident.
> Terminally ill with a life expectancy of six months or less.
> Capable of making and communicating health care decisions for yourself.

To obtain life-ending medication, patients must make two oral requests to their physicians that are at least fifteen days apart and one written request. Only currently licensed doctors of medicine or osteopathy may write lethal prescriptions.

The physician must certify that the patient is terminally ill and has six months or less to live, and that diagnosis must be certified by a consulting physician, who must also certify that the patient is mentally competent to make and communicate health care decisions. Physicians also must inform patients of alternatives, including palliative care, hospice, and pain-management options.

In Oregon and Washington, physicians must encourage patients, but not require them, to notify their next of kin about their prescription request. In the debate about aid in dying, proponents see many of these rules as overly burdensome, whereas opponents worry that there are not enough safeguards.

Again, if you are considering aid in dying, talk with your doctor and your loved ones. Know that we can do a great deal to reduce suffering and address the concerns that led you to pursue aid in dying. Know *all* your options.

AFTER DEATH

Right after a loved one dies, it's common to feel numb, disoriented, and stunned. Even when you are expecting it, a loved one's death can feel like a surprise and can hit you hard. Responses also vary from culture to culture. Mourners in some cultures loudly wail and scream, while those in others react stoically and silently. Different cultures have different customs, rituals, and procedures. They may cleanse, prepare, dress, and deal with bodies differently.

Many families don't know what to do when a loved one dies. An expected death at the end of serious illness is not an emergency. Take your time, allow yourself to react, and don't suppress your emotions. It's fine to spend time with your loved one who has just died. If your loved one died at home, call your doctor, hospice, or home care agency. If they died in a hospital, tell a nurse. If you want certain rituals followed, make your wishes clear and, if possible, tell the nurse and doctor in advance.

> Many of our Buddhist patients ask us not to move the deceased's body for several hours after death. They believe that soon after death, the soul leaves the body for the next life, so it's important not to disturb the body because it could confuse the soul. When we know families' wishes, we can plan ahead and make sure we respect them.

Follow your loved one's wishes. Respect his or her beliefs and traditions. If your loved one was part of a religious community, inform his or her clergyman of your loved one's death. It can be hard to inform others about your loved one's death, to have to say it over and over, so enlist others who can perform that task.

Recognize that after your loved one dies, you'll be filled with grief. Deep, painful sorrow may envelop you, but then you'll also have moments of calm and even joy remembering happier times. Your emotions will vary. They may not be strong, uniform, and consistent all the time. Instead, they may move from extreme to extreme and everywhere in between.

Telling the story—sharing what happened with your loved one's illness and his or her end-of-life experience—can be cathartic and provide a much-needed emotional release. It can help you deal with your sorrow and grief. If someone you know is ill or has died, ask about it because it can help his or her family to talk about it. There is power in telling; it's important to tell and to listen.

Grief can be hyperacute, but after about six months it tends to ease. If, after six months, you continue to have intrusive thoughts or disturbing dreams and you are crying and blue, seek professional help. You won't ever get over your grief—you'll always miss your loved one—but the intensity and pain of your sadness should fade over time.

Times of death are not times to be alone. Be with others. If you need to, take time off. I'm often surprised when people go back to work the day after a loved one's death. The Jewish religion mandates seven days of mourning after a close loved one has died. It's called sitting shiva, (*shiva* means "seven)." During that time, family and friends visit the survivors and pay their respects. It's considered a holy act to visit the bereaved and to bring food.

Even if your tradition doesn't mandate it, being with others is important, as is taking time to grieve. Take time off of work, even if it's just a few days. Invite people to be with you. When you're grieving, support groups and professional help can be extremely beneficial. Hospices offer this help regardless of whether your loved one used their services.

RX

Death is sad. It's filled with grief and loss. Too often the medical care provided makes the end of life more painful than it needs to be and compounds grief. Try to be prepared; try to anticipate when the end is near. Being prepared can ease the suffering of both those who are about to die and their loved ones. When death is at hand, disconnect the monitors, turn off the machines, stop the poking and prodding, and focus on being together and on comfort, dignity, gratitude, and love.

Loved ones remember the end of life. That memory will always be sad, but it doesn't have to be complicated by resentment, guilt, and regret. Let medical care support you and your loved one but not detract from this profound, natural, and indelible event.

FINAL THOUGHTS

WE DREAD THE MOMENT WHEN WE GET BAD NEWS.
Learning that we're seriously ill is an affront to our sense of order
in the world. It feels unfair, and it is. It challenges every aspect
of our lives, our relationships, self-image, work, religion, beliefs,
attitudes, expectations, hopes, and fears.

When you're seriously ill, the future, which seemed infinite,
is now limited. Even though you rationally know that each life
has to end, that fact is easy to forget. In many ways, you need to
forget in order to face each day. Serious illness forces you to face
your mortality. Life after the diagnosis is challenging and frightening. The possibility of being cured means there is a possibility
of not being cured.

Most of us will get bad news. We'll feel its crushing weight.
It can feel like a blow to the gut that takes our breath away. We
probably won't hear anything after we get the news, though in all
likelihood, our doctor will talk about treatment plans. If you're

reading this book, it is likely that you or your loved one is already living with serious illness. The challenge, and the focus of this book, is how best to embrace life after the diagnosis.

First, know that you don't have to, and should not, face life after the diagnosis alone. It takes a village—so gather the villagers. Your family, friends, caregivers, doctors, nurses, social workers, and others will form the team that will help you move through your illness.

Second, remember that you're the chief of the village. You're the decision maker. It's your life, and it's your body that will undergo treatment. Get the information you need to make the most informed decisions. Don't accept evasive answers, platitudes, or generalities. Understand what doctors say, ask them what they really mean, and use the information to make the decisions that are best for you. Your doctors and nurses want to help. Be an active part of your team. Help them help you.

Expect to have times—many times—when you feel like you're between a rock and a hard place with no easy, obvious, or good escape routes. Know that there is no right or wrong treatment and no good or bad treatment. When you have to decide which treatments to undergo, the answers may be elusive because each serious illness, each case, is unique. The price of pursuing all treatments at any cost can be steep—and often, less is more. Treatments that you take to help you live longer may not actually help you live any longer. As you get sicker, they may even make your life shorter and ruin the life you hoped to extend.

Remember, you always have a choice. Find the path that is right for you and that achieves the right balance. Let your values and goals guide you. Ultimately, it's not about the treatments but what the treatments will help you achieve.

SERIOUS ILLNESS STINKS

I've cared for thousands of people with serious illness and have seen the devastation and havoc serious illness wreaks. There's no way around it: serious illness stinks. If it were up to me, we wouldn't experience serious illness. We would live to be very old, with all of our faculties intact, and one night, we would die peacefully in our sleep.

My Safta used to sign birthday cards with the wish that you should live to 120. Moses lived 120 years. A traditional birthday wish is that you should have a long life like Moses, the greatest teacher and leader of the Jewish people. But as she got older, my grandmother changed it a bit. In Hebrew, she switched just one letter, and the change in meaning was profound. Rather than saying, "Live to one hundred *and* twenty," she said, "Live to one hundred *like* twenty."

Live long and live well. My Safta understood that a good life is even more important than a long life. She lived that saying and declined chemotherapy when she was diagnosed with lung cancer at age ninety-three. Not all of us will live that long, but we can all live the essence of that saying by living well.

The challenge we face is to live as well as possible with serious illness. I've learned that we can meet this challenge. Serious illness doesn't have to ruin your life or shut it down. Even in what feels like a tragedy, you can still have great joy along with the sadness. You can find great opportunities to achieve important goals even if the time is short.

The key is to face serious illness and the possibility of death head on. Hiding will not make it go away, but it may lead you down a path that will make the quality of your life worse and your life span shorter. The fact that time is limited puts a premium on making the most of the time we have left. It compels us to make the most of each day. While all of us may understand this intellectually, those who are seriously ill feel it every day.

LANGUAGE OF THE HEART

In my work, I find great inspiration in poetry because it speaks the language of the heart. I especially love reading Mary Oliver, whom I call the poet laureate of palliative care. She ends her poem "The Summer Day" by asking, "Tell me, what is it you plan to do / with your one wild and precious life?" This is the essential question that serious illness makes urgent. It's one of the most important questions any of us will ever have to answer and the reason I wrote this book—to help people with serious illness make the most of their life after the diagnosis.

Think about how you want to *live* with serious illness. Life after the diagnosis is the rest of your life. *Living* as well as possible with serious illness is the most important thing you can do. Focusing on how you want to die will not guarantee that you'll live the way you want, but living every day according to your values and goals will help the end unfold in the way you hope.

Much has been written about helping people achieve a good death. That's not my goal for two reasons. First, my focus is not on dying well, but on living well with serious illness. I strive to help patients who are dying be comfortable, be at peace, and have their dignity intact. Second, I don't believe good deaths exist. As my colleague Sharon Sutton once said, "The only good death is someone else's."

Death may be a relief from a long decline. It may come at the end of a long life well lived. We may be able to understand it and accept it. That doesn't make it good. Death is always filled with loss, sadness, and grief, which is why death isn't good. And the more we have lived well and loved deeply, the harder and sadder death will be.

Death can also be peaceful, comfortable, and dignified, and that's better than a death with pain, discomfort, and a loss of dignity, but it's still not good. Too often medical care makes the end of life worse than it needs to be; it puts people through needless pain, misery, and humiliation. My goal is to help my patients live well and have a better end of life than they would have without medical care.

> Imagine life as an airplane flight. To take off, we need a lot of help from the crew—just as at birth we need help from medical professionals. When we're airborne, the flight is smooth, until we hit bumps and turbulence. Some bumps are big and scary, so the crew has to act quickly. Eventually, each flight must end.
>
> In medicine and life, we frequently don't acknowledge that the flight will soon be over and we'll have to land. We think we can stay in the sky forever, even when three of our four engines are shot and the fourth is sputtering. To make matters worse, most doctors and nurses don't know how to land, so as the last engine is failing, they're desperately trying to keep the plane aloft.
>
> Often, when we push too hard and refuse to give up, our lives crash and burn onto the runway. Wouldn't it be better if the passengers and crew understood that the plane had to land because the engines were giving out? We could bring the plane down smoothly and gently and touch down softly. The flight would end without panic and fear. That's my goal in writing this book: to help you have a smooth approach and to touch down gently and peacefully. You can't land gently unless you prepare.

I love medicine. I love the treatments that help cure disease and help people live better. When I was a medical student and resident, AIDS was a new scourge that was killing many young men in their prime. We had an entire ward at San Francisco General Hospital dedicated to caring for AIDS patients. It's where I learned palliative care, though we didn't have a name for it then. Today, that ward no longer exists. AIDS continues to be a chronic illness, but in the United States, people with AIDS usually die from something else. I love that in my lifetime, we turned a universally fatal disease into a chronic disease. I hope to see many more such transformations.

Modern medicine is remarkable. But too often promises are made that cannot be kept. The media is filled with ads for cancer centers that promise cures even when the reality is that in the United States, cancer is the second leading cause of death. When we're sick and suffering, we hope that we'll be cured, but in pursuit of that hope we often ruin the very life we hope to save and squander the time we have.

As a patient with cancer once told me, "You know, Dr. Pantilat, I have cancer that will take my life, but you could get hit by a bus walking to your car and die today." I was struck by his comment, by the reminder that while my patient knew that his tomorrows were limited, mine were too. We're in this together.

Tomorrow is not guaranteed. Life after the diagnosis will be the hardest time of your life, but it will also offer opportunities and meaning. Focus on them. Find balance in treatments. Choose your path carefully. Stay true to your values and goals. Get help, have hope, love fully. Make the most of each day, whether you think you'll have many more or only a few. Live well during your one wild and precious life.

APPENDIX A

Evidence

PALLIATIVE CARE STUDIES AND PAPERS

THE FOLLOWING ARE SOME OF THE MOST IMPORTANT STUDIES AND PAPERS that have reported the benefits of palliative care. If you're interested in understanding more about the evidence for palliative care, read them. And, by the way, you should seek similar evidence for any medical intervention you agree to in order to understand the risks and benefits of each.

CHAPTER 2

2.1 **Multidisciplinary care for people with ALS.** Van den Berg JP, Kalmijn S, Lindeman E, et al. *Multidisciplinary ALS care improves quality of life in patients with ALS. Neurology.* 2005;65(8):1264–1267.

2.2 **Palliative care helps you live better and longer.** Temel JS, Greer JA, Muzikansky A, et al. *Early palliative care for patients with metastatic non-small-cell lung cancer. N Engl J Med.* 2010;363(8):733–742. This rigorously designed, three-year study led by Dr. Jennifer Temel, conducted from 2006–2009, and published in the *New England Journal of Medicine* in 2010, is a landmark study in palliative care. If you read only one study, read this one.

This study involved 151 people who were recently diagnosed with incurable lung cancer, which means that it had spread outside their lungs and, even with the best treatment, could not be cured. On average, patients with this condition, including those who go through the most advanced treatments, live for about nine months after their initial diagnosis. Every patient in the study received the best oncology treatments at Massachusetts General Hospital, an affiliate of Harvard University. Half of the patients studied were randomly selected to also receive palliative care. The study found that the patients who got palliative care along with their cancer treatments had less pain, less shortness of breath, less depression, happier lives, and a better quality of life, and they lived longer by 2.7 months—living nearly a year compared to nine months for those who didn't receive palliative care. And the patients who received palliative care had no harmful side effects from it. That means that palliative care was as good as, or better than, chemotherapy in helping people feel better and live longer.

Palliative care, when provided along with chemotherapy and other cancer treatments, helped people feel better and live longer with no side effects. For those of us who work in palliative care, the findings of this study came as no surprise. We see similar results all the time.

CHAPTER 3

3.1 **Chemotherapy use in the last six months of life does not improve quality of life or extend life.** Prigerson HG, Bao Y, Shah MA, et al. *Chemotherapy Use, Performance Status, and Quality of Life at the End of Life. JAMA Oncol.* 2015;1(6):778–784. For people with advanced cancer, chemotherapy is given to improve quality of life and extend life. This study sought to examine if these goals are achieved. The study enrolled patients with metastatic cancer at six cancer centers across the country. The researchers measured quality of life at baseline when people enrolled and then followed them until they died. The researchers recorded whether people received chemotherapy and asked the surviving loved one to rate the patient's quality of life near the end of life.

For people with the best quality of life at baseline, chemotherapy use was associated with worse quality of life near the end of life. For those with worse quality of life at baseline, chemotherapy use did not make it better or worse. Regardless of baseline quality of life, there was no difference in survival between those who received chemotherapy and those who did not. Of course, it can be difficult to know precisely when you have only six months to live, but your doctor can make a good guess (see chapter 4). The point is that when you are very sick with metastatic cancer, chemotherapy is unlikely to help you live better or longer. The study was completed in 2008, and new treatments for cancer, including immunotherapy and biologic agents, are being discovered all the time. Will these treatments fundamentally change this story? We hope so. But the jury is still out. In the meantime, be skeptical and ask a lot of questions.

3.2 **Dialysis does not help sick nursing home patients become more functional.** Kurella TM, Covinsky KE, Chertow GM, Yaffe K, Landefeld CS, McCulloch CE. *Functional status of elderly adults before and after initiation of dialysis. N Engl J Med.* 2009;361(16):1539–1547. This study analyzed data on over 3,700 people with kidney disease living in nursing homes who started dialysis over a two-year period between 1998 and 2000. The researchers found that starting dialysis was associated with a worsening in patients's functional capabilities. They also learned that one year after starting dialysis only 13 percent of patients had maintained their ability to function at the same level, and 60 percent had died.

CHAPTER 5

5.1 **Communication between patients and doctors.** Beckman HB, Frankel RM. *The effect of physician behavior on the collection of data. Ann Intern Med.* 1984;101(5):692–696. This was one of the first studies to examine how patients and doctors communicate. The researchers audio-recorded patient-doctor visits and analyzed the tape recordings. From these, they learned that doctors interrupted patients, on average, after only eighteen seconds.

That is a very short time to talk about important issues. In nearly 70 percent of visits, the doctor interrupted the patient's very first statement, and only once out of fifty visits did the patient get back to that topic.

CHAPTER 6

6.1 **There is no consistent association between MRI findings and back pain.** Savage RA, Whitehouse GH, Roberts N. *The relationship between the magnetic resonance imaging appearance of the lumbar spine and low back pain, age and occupation in males. Eur Spine* 1997;6(2):106–114.

6.2 **Assessing pain in patients with dementia.** Zwakhalen SM, Hamers JP, Abu-Saad HH, Berger MP. *Pain in elderly people with severe dementia: a systematic review of behavioural pain assessment tools. BMC Geriatr.* 2006;6:3. An excellent review of different instruments used to assess pain in patients with dementia, with recommendations for which ones to use.

CHAPTER 7

7.1 **Exercise as treatment for depression.** Kvam S, Kleppe CL, Nordhus IH, Hovland A. *Exercise as a treatment for depression: A meta-analysis. J Affect Disord.* 2016;202:67–86. Exercise works to treat depression and can be effective in combination with medications.

7.2 **Californians' attitudes about death and dying.** http://www.chcf.org /publications/2012/02/final-chapter-death-dying. California may be a bit different than the rest of the United States, but people are people. This survey of 1,669 Californians, including 393 who had a loved one who died in the preceding year, sheds light on attitudes toward serious illness and care at the end of life.

CHAPTER 8

8.1 **Impact of hospice on spouses.** Christakis NA, Iwashyna TJ. *The health impact of health care on families: a matched cohort study of hospice use by decedents and mortality outcomes in surviving, widowed spouses. Soc Sci Med.* 2003;57(3):465–475. This study used a large database to examine whether hospice use impacts mortality of spouses. The researchers compared bereaved spouses of patients who received hospice care with those who did not and found that, especially for bereaved wives, there was a significant decrease in the risk of death for those whose spouse used hospice services.

CHAPTER 9

9.1 **Chemotherapy use in the last six months of life does not improve quality of life or extend life.** Prigerson HG, Bao Y, Shah MA, et al. *Chemotherapy Use, Performance Status, and Quality of Life at the End of Life. JAMA Oncol.* 2015;1(6):778–784. (see 3.1)

9.2 **Palliative care helps you live better and longer.** Temel JS, Greer JA, Muzikansky A, et al. *Early palliative care for patients with metastatic non-small-cell lung cancer. N Engl J Med.* 2010;363(8):733–742. (see 2.2)

CHAPTER 10

10.1 **Quality of life is hard to judge for others.** Brickman P, Coates D, Janoff-Bulman R. *Lottery winners and accident victims: is happiness relative? J Pers Soc Psychol.* 1978;36(8):917–927. Researchers investigated quality of life of lottery winners compared with that of people paralyzed after an accident. They found that those who were paralyzed were not quite as happy as the lottery winners, but the difference was small. And people in both groups found about the same amount of happiness from everyday experiences like talking with friends, and they reported that they would be happy in the future in equal measure.

CHAPTER 11

11.1 **Californians' attitudes about their wishes for care at the end of life.** http://www.chcf.org/publications/2012/02/final-chapter -death-dying. (see 7.2)

11.2 **CPR on television.** *Miracles and misinformation.* Diem SJ, Lantos JD, Tulsky JA. *N Engl J Med.* 1996;334(24):1578–1582. CPR on television is very different from CPR in real life. On television CPR cases is rarely performed on older patients; in the real world the majority of people who undergo the procedure are older. On television most CPR is done for acute injury; in real life most CPR is done for underlying heart disease. Most important, whereas on television 75 percent of people survive and two-thirds do well, in real life about one-third of people survive the CPR episode and about a third of those leave the hospital. The lesson is that you should not base your decision about CPR on what you've seen on television, but rather get accurate information from your doctor and nurse.

CHAPTER 12

12.1 **If palliative care was a pill, everyone would take it.** Pantilat SZ. *When it's the right care, more is better. Arch Intern Med.* 2012:3–4. A commentary on two cases of patients who needed and received palliative care that reflects on how common and widely used palliative care would be if it were as simple to get as a prescription.

12.2 **Palliative care conversations improve care for patients and their families.** Wright AA, Zhang B, Ray A, et al. *Associations between end-of-life discussions, patient mental health, medical care near death, and caregiver bereavement adjustment. JAMA.* 2008;300(14):1665–1673. Patients with incurable, metastatic cancer were studied at seven sites around the country from 2002 to 2008. The study, which followed the participants until they died, asked one question: "Have you and your doctor had any discussions about the kind of care you would like to receive if you were approaching the end of your life?" Holding these discussions is a centerpiece of palliative care, and we refer to them as "palliative care conversations."

Overall, 37 percent of those studied had palliative care conversations. Interestingly, that number varied from 16 percent at one site to 61 percent at another. The likelihood of having this conversation depended on where the patients received care. The patients who had palliative care conversations with their doctors (1) had a better quality of life at the end of their lives and (2) were less likely to receive care in an ICU, to be intubated, or to have CPR at the end of their lives.

The study also followed the participants' survivors and interviewed them six months after the participants died. The survivors of the patients who had palliative care conversations with their doctor had better health and quality of life and were less likely to have depression six months later. This study is remarkable because it showed that palliative care conversations are not just good for the patients who have them, they are also good for their loved ones. Few treatments improve the health of the patient treated *and* that of their loved ones. Certainly surgery, chemotherapy, and radiation do not. The only other treatment I can think of that helps patients and others is quitting smoking; it improves the health of the smoker, their family members, and everyone around them.

12.3 **Palliative care helps you live better and longer.** Temel JS, Greer JA, Muzikansky A, et al. *Early palliative care for patients with metastatic non-small-cell lung cancer. N Engl J Med.* 2010;363(8):733–742. (see 2.2)

12.4 **Palliative care in the hospital.** Gade G, Venohr I, Conner D, et al. *Impact of an inpatient palliative care team: a randomized control trial. J Palliat Med.* 2008;11(2):180–190. This study enrolled hospitalized patients who were seriously ill and whose physicians said that they would not have been surprised if the patients died in the next year. While the physicians' statements may not seem precise, the answer to the "surprise question" is a pretty good way to find those who need palliative care. The patients who agreed to participate were randomly assigned to receive palliative care in the hospital and after discharge in an office or at home. The researchers found that patients who received palliative care didn't live longer or shorter, but they lived better. They were more satisfied with their care, more likely to complete an advance health care directive, and, if they were admitted to the hospital, were less likely to spend time in the ICU.

12.5 **Palliative care conversations improve care for patients and their families.** Wright AA, Zhang B, Ray A, et al. *Associations between end-of-life discussions, patient mental health, medical care near death, and caregiver bereavement adjustment. JAMA.* 2008;300(14):1665–1673. (see 12.2)

12.6 **Surviving spouses of patients who use hospice are less likely to die in the eighteen months following the death of their loved one.** Christakis NA, Iwashyna TJ. *The health impact of health care on families: a matched cohort study of hospice use by decedents and mortality outcomes in surviving, widowed spouses. Soc Sci Med.* 2003;57(3):465–475. Wives of men who used hospice services were less likely to die in the eighteen months after the death of their husbands than wives of men who did not use hospice. The benefit in life span is similar to or better than that from many lifestyle modifications promoted to improve health. (see 8.1)

12.7 **Oncology society endorses palliative care for all patients with metastatic cancer.** Smith TJ, Temin S, Alesi ER, et al. *American Society of Clinical Oncology provisional clinical opinion: the integration of palliative care into standard oncology care. J Clin Oncol.* 2012;30(8):880–887. The American Society of Clinical Oncology is the largest professional organization of cancer doctors in the world. The society convened a group of experts to review the research and found that palliative care provided along with cancer care improved symptoms, improved quality of life, and increased satisfaction with care and was also beneficial to caregivers. The panel also noted that there has never been a study that found harm from palliative care. Based on this sound scientific evidence, the expert panel recommended that all patients with metastatic cancer receive palliative care.

12.8 **Californians' attitudes about their wishes for care at the end of life.** http://www.chcf.org/publications/2012/02/final-chapter -death-dying. (see 7.2)

CHAPTER 13

13.1 **Statistics about hospice care in the United States from the National Hospice and Palliative Care Organization.** http://www .nhpco.org/hospice-statistics-research-press-room/facts-hospice -and-palliative-care.

13.2 **Hospice care for more than seven days improves quality of life at the end of life.** Wright AA, Zhang B, Ray A, et al. *Associations between end-of-life discussions, patient mental health, medical* *care near death, and caregiver bereavement adjustment. JAMA.* 2008;300(14):1665–1673. Patients who received hospice care for seven days or less had the same quality of life at the end of life as those patients who received no hospice care. Those who received hospice care for more than two months had a significantly higher quality of life at the end of life. Longer hospice stays are better. Don't put off enrolling.

CHAPTER 14

14.1 **Access to interpreters in health care.** Youdelman MK. *The medical tongue: U.S. laws and policies on language access. Health Aff (Millwood).* 2008;27(2):424–433. The federal government and all fifty states mandate access to interpreters for patients with limited English proficiency in all health care settings.

CHAPTER 15

15.1 **Artificial nutrition does not improve outcomes for people with advanced serious illness.** Koretz RL, Avenell A, Lipman TO, Braunschweig CL, Milne AC. *Does enteral nutrition affect clinical outcome? A systematic review of the randomized trials. Am J Gastroenterol.* 2007;102(2):412–429. This paper reviewed rigorously designed, published studies and found no evidence supporting the use of artificial nutrition for people with advanced serious illness.

ACKNOWLEDGMENTS

THERE ARE MANY PEOPLE I WANT TO THANK FOR HELPING THIS BOOK COME to be. Medicine is called a practice because doctors are always learning and honing our craft. In my twenty-seven years as a physician I have had the distinct pleasure and honor to work with, care for, and learn from many wonderful patients, colleagues, mentors, students, and teachers, and all of them are in one way or another in this book. If I forget to thank someone, I hope you will forgive the unintentional oversight.

The idea for this book came over a decade ago from talking with the late Phil Lawrence, the father of a dear friend, whose wife was living with advanced cancer. Phil's daughter Joanne asked if I would talk with her dad about decisions he and his wife were facing and what to expect as she got sicker. I wasn't sure that a phone call to the husband of someone I wasn't directly caring for would be that helpful, but it turned out it was. I thank Phil and Joanne for thinking that I could be helpful and for planting the seed of the book.

I became a palliative care physician before it was even a medical specialty and have learned so much from so many. When I was a medical student at UCSF, there was no palliative care service. We saw the need and decided to fill it. I especially want to thank Stephen McPhee, Jane Hirsch, and Carol Mowbray for their partnership, support, and vision that led us together to found the palliative care service at UCSF, as well as Tom Bookwalter, Jane Hawgood, Mike Rabow, and Rod Seeger, who helped build it. I also want to thank my chairman at the time, Lee Goldman, for supporting my interest. Special thanks to my dean and former chairman of medicine Talmadge King, who has been a steadfast supporter and a kind and insightful mentor, leader, and role model. Special thanks also to Bob Wachter, my division chief and friend, who created a welcoming and supportive home for palliative care in hospital medicine and who by example as a leader, mentor, and author inspired me to write this book. I also want to thank my colleagues in the Division of Hospital Medicine at UCSF who have embraced the palliative care program and my many friends and colleagues at the Society of Hospital Medicine, especially Larry Wellikson, who have supported and promoted palliative care as a core part of hospital medicine.

I want to thank the many leaders at UCSF who have supported the palliative care program: Sam Hawgood, Mark Laret, Ken Jones, Josh Adler, Sheila Antrum, Tomi Ryba, Barrie Strickland, Adrienne Green, Jay Harris, Kevin Grumbach, Susan Smith, Colleen Kilvahan, and David Vlahov. I have spent my entire career at UCSF, and it has been a remarkable professional home. The depth and breadth of talent at UCSF is amazing, and I am grateful for the many opportunities it has afforded me.

I have also had the great fortune to know many dedicated and committed people who share our vision of what care can and should be for people with serious illness and who have supported our innovative programs and ideas. Special thanks to my dear friends Alan Kates and the late John Burnard, who embraced palliative care even before it had a name. Together they have done so much to enshrine palliative care at UCSF. We couldn't have gotten here without your help. Special thanks also to the Hellman Family Foundation, especially Trisha Hellman Gibbs and Judith Hellman; your support means so much. Special thanks to the Alafi Family Foundation for their steadfast support over the years. Thanks also to Bill and Deborah Harlan for your support and your example of the continual pursuit of excellence.

Palliative care is provided by a team, and I have had the extreme good fortune to work with so many compassionate, caring, and bright clinicians from so many disciplines and from whom I have learned so much. I want to thank our wonderful palliative care team at UCSF: Denah Joseph, Laura Woods, Bridget Sumser, Susan Barbour, Wendy Anderson, Tom Reid, Kara Bischoff, Kana McKee, Brook Calton, Dawn Gross, Giovanni Elia, Marcia Glass, Mike Rabow, Sarah Adkins, Nancy Shepard Lopez, and Daphne Stuart. I also want to thank my outstanding research team: David O'Riordan, Teri Rose, Angela Marks, Shayna McElveny, Rachel Stone, and Alex Rantes. You are more than colleagues; you are friends, family, and teachers. You make it fun to come to work every day.

At UCSF I am blessed to have so many outstanding colleagues as partners in promoting palliative care across our institution: Mike Rabow, Christine Ritchie, Rebecca Sudore, Sharon Kaufman, Niraj Sehgal, Anne Kinderman, Heather Harris, Maya Katz, Teresa DeMarco, Louise Walter, Doranne Donesky, Kathleen Puntillo, Alex Smith, Eric Widera, Ami Parekh, Lynn Flint, Olivia Herbert, Suzy Beemer, and Susan Penney. I also want to thank the hundreds of dedicated palliative care professionals from across the country and around the world that I have had the pleasure to work with through the Palliative Care Quality Network and our Palliative Care Leadership Center.

I am extremely fortunate to have wonderful mentors, colleagues, students, and mentees who have been generous with their time and ideas. You will see many of our conversations reflected in this book. Special thanks to Kathy Foley for your kindness and your belief in me; Betty Ferrell, Randy Curtis, Trish Davidson, Kathy Dracup, Christine Ritchie, Jean Kutner, and James Tulsky—our conversation on the way to Granlibakken provided great insights about our work; Susan Block, Andy Billings, Bernie Lo, Diane Meier, Sean Morrison, Amy Abernethy, Ira Byock, Karl Lorenz, Bob Arnold, Jeff Burack, David Currow, Tony Back, Irene Higginson, Lucy Selman, Carol Douglas, Charles von Gunten, Frank Ferris, Dan Lowenstein, Judy Thomas, Peter Lindenauer, Molly Bourne, Toby Campbell, Arif Kamal, Janet Bull, Claire Creutzfeldt, Rachel Adams, Rachelle Bernacki, Vanessa Grubbs, Chris Pietras, and Daniel Lam. Thank you for your friendship and partnership.

I also want to thank my many friends outside of my professional world who have been a great support in writing this book. Special thanks to Tony—our breakfasts in Burlingame make my life richer and help me know what it is to live well—Soo, Ari, Kristin, Mike, Bao, Tim, Danny, Linda, Robert, Lisa, Laurel, Dean, Ariella, Trish, Randy, Lloyd, and Jill.

Over the years I have enjoyed support from many foundations that share a vision for helping people live well with serious illness. Thanks to the Soros Foundation and the Project on Death in America, which helped me become and see myself as a palliative care physician; the Robert Wood Johnson Foundation, especially Steve Schroeder and Rosemary Gibson—thanks for making so much lemonade from lemons; the California Health Care Foundation, especially Kate O'Malley, my colleague, friend, and visionary, as well as Mark Smith, Sophia Chang, and Kelly Pfeifer—the impact of your support is enormous; the Archstone Foundation, especially Joseph Prevratil, Mary Ellen Kullman, Laura Rath, Tanisha Davis, and Thomas Brewer; the UniHealth Foundation, especially Mary Odell—thank you for supporting so much palliative care; the Irvine Foundation; the Kettering Family Foundation, especially Lisa and Charlie for your belief in our work; the JEHT Foundation; and the Cambia Foundation, especially Mark Ganz, Peggy Maguire, Angela Hult, Jennifer Fuller, and Elyse Salend—thank you for your friendship, partnership, and vision and for walking the walk together: the future of palliative care is secure with your help.

I also thank my many patients and their families who have faced serious illness with courage and allowed me to walk with them on their difficult journey. I have learned so much from you about medicine, about the sacred trust of being a physician, about the agony of making difficult decisions, and about what makes life worth living. Special thanks to the family members who make up our Palliative Care Patient and Family Advisory Council: Ann Berkey, Trisha Hellman Gibbs, Alan Kates, Joe Bertain, Kai Yee Woo, Jordan Goldstein, and David Broom.

The idea for this book grew out of experiences of helping friends, family, and colleagues with serious illness. It was during my sabbatical as a Fulbright scholar in Sydney, Australia, in 2007–08, while riding the 378 bus from Bronte to Railway Square that I first outlined the chapters for what would ultimately become this book. That table of contents might have stayed just that if it were not for my coach and friend Phil Glosserman, who has been a steady voice urging me to just "write the book." Like any good coach, Phil has provided the right balance of kindness and toughness, holding me to deadlines and keeping me on track. Thank you, Phil. This book would not have come to be without you. Thanks also to Stephen Purcell for his ongoing encouragement and support.

Thanks also to friends who read early chapters and provided detailed feedback. My late dear friend Bo Burt provided great insights on the voice and approach. Many thanks to Robert Sapolsky, Bob Wachter, and Katie Hafner, who provided helpful feedback on an early draft. Thanks to David Casarett, Angelo Volandes, Chuck Ryan, Bob Wachter, Louise Aronson, and Ira Byock for sharing their experiences and insights as physician-writers. It has indeed been a labor of love. Thanks to Cam Sutter for valuable input on caring for children of adults with serious illness and to Molly Bourne for great insights and input on the chapter about hospice. Thanks also to Denah Joseph, Laura Woods, and Bridget Sumser for your insights into the practical, caregiving, and spiritual aspects of serious illness.

Writing is largely a solitary affair, and the blank page can be very daunting. When I started writing this book in earnest over three years ago, I knew I wanted to work with an editor, as I had done for other important projects in the past. I was fortunate to meet and work with Mark Steisel. I offer my sincere and deepest gratitude to Mark, who has been my partner in writing this book. He has taken my outline, ideas, and stories and helped me craft them into a book. Mark has helped with editing and getting my ideas onto the page and has also been an audience for the tone and content. It has been a great pleasure to work with you.

I want to thank my agent, John Willig, whose enthusiasm and excitement about my book reignited my own. John helped to shape the proposal into one that captured the content and purpose of my book, and he found a publisher, Dan Ambrosio at Da Capo Lifelong Books, who was equally enthusiastic about it. Dan and his team at Da Capo have been a joy to work with—supportive, collaborative, and helpful at every turn. Thank you.

In this book I write about my family and the experiences of my parents, Sara and Yoav, my mother-in-law, Shirley, and father-in-law, Ray, and my grandparents, my Saba and Safta. I come to this topic not just as a doctor, but as a son, grandson, family member, and friend who has experienced loss and grief. I learned a great deal about illness and dying from my family and much more about how to be a good person, live a good and meaningful life, and leave a legacy of goodness. May their memories be a blessing. Special thanks and love to my wonderful sisters, Tammy and Dana, for your love and support and for being with Mom every day through her illness. You provided her, and me, great comfort. Special thanks and love to my aunt, Ayala, who taught me more about caregiving than any book or paper ever could. Your care is exactly what any of us could hope for when dealing with serious illness. Thanks and love to my uncle Dennis for a lifetime of support—from that very first paper airplane. Thanks to my brother-in-law David Fenton, whose pursuit of excellence has been a great source of inspiration, and to my extended family Darren, Jodi, Larry, and Mark for your encouragement and support.

Finally, I want to thank my amazing family. My children, Yoav, Ben, and Adam, remind me every day about the joy and meaning of life. Your hard work and perseverance have helped to motivate me during the long hours of writing. Thanks for all the laughter, adventures, and *nachas*. I give my deepest thanks and gratitude to my wife, Cindy. I love you. You are a constant and unwavering source of love and support. You keep me honest, help me see with clarity, and make it possible to pursue the work I love. Your example of a dedicated, loving, and engaged partner, parent, and physician is a model and a source of inspiration to me. You are an amazing life partner, and I am so grateful to be able to share so much joy, and occasional sadness, together. I look forward to growing old together.

Steven Z. Pantilat, MD
San Francisco, CA
July 2016

INDEX